CCM Certification Made Easy

3rd Edition

Deanna Cooper Gillingham, RN, CCM

Copyright © 2020 Deanna Cooper Gillingham

To request permission, contact the publisher at Support@CaseManagementInstitute.com

ISBN Paperback: 978-1-943889-14-3

Library of Congress Control Number: 2020912947

First paperback edition December 2014, 2nd Ed. July 2016, Revised 2nd Ed. July 2019.

Edited by Rachael Flug

Cover art by Abigail Gusto

Layout by Abigail Gusto

Excerpt from CMSA's Standards of Practice for Case Managers reprinted with permission, the Case Management Society of America, 6301 Ranch Drive, Little Rock, AR 72223, www.cmsa.org.

Blue Bayou Press, LLC

5753 Highway 85N #4010
Crestview, FL 32536

BlueBayouPress.com
CaseManagementInstitute.com

DEDICATION

This book is dedicated to the following people, without whom I would not be who I am today and the book would not have been possible.

Brenda El Dada who saw a great case manager in me, and took a chance on me before I even understood what a case manager was.

Martha Pressley-Turner who mentored me from a nurse into a great case manager and continues to be a friend and mentor.

The Case Managers Community FB Group whose encouragement and support to each other and to me, as well as their dedication to their clients, is inspiring.

Abi Carmen who is my partner in everything. He keeps me focused on the priorities, and makes me write even when I don't want to. His belief in me gives me the confidence I need to succeed and for that, I am beyond grateful.

ACKNOWLEDGEMENTS

A book covering as many topics as this one does is not the work of one person. It takes a team of experts dedicated to the growth and development of professional case managers to create a comprehensive work such as this. I am humbled and honored to have such a dedicated team enthusiastic to be a part of this endeavor.

First, I would like to thank Colleen Morley, DNP, RN, CCM, CMAC, CMCN, ACM-RN for her contributions to the chapter on Quality. She filled in the gaps by writing content and was a valuable consultant and content editor. Her knowledge and expertise, as well as willingness to put up with me through numerous rewrites mean more to me than words can express.

I owe an enormous debt of gratitude to those who helped me to write the Test Your Knowledge questions. This job is at the top of my list of least favorite things to do. After years of requests for this feature in the book, it finally came to fruition thanks to Ellen Fink-Samnick, MSW, ACSW, LCSW, CCM, CRP; Carol King, MSN, RN-BC; Barbara Kuritz, RN, BS, LHCA, CCM; Anne Llewellyn, MS, BHSA, RN-BC, CCM, CRRN; and Laura Ostrowsky, RN, CCM, MUP.

In addition to writing the Test Your Knowledge questions, Ellen Fink-Samnick and Anne Llewellyn had additional roles. Ellen was a consultant and content editor to the Ethics Chapter and gave me detailed and constructive comments on that chapter. Anne has been an essential contributor since the 2nd edition where she graciously accepted the role of a content editor.

I would also like to thank Meredith Ximines-Mullings, MSN, RN, CEN for her assistance as a content editor and consultant for the sections on Insurance Principles. She gave freely of her time to give constructive comments and specific recommendations to clarify concepts while explaining the rationale for those recommendations.

Contents

Contents

Contents

Contents

Psychosocial Concepts and Support Systems   133

Contents

Contents

Contents

Ethical, Legal, and Practice Standards   263

Contents

Introduction

Congratulations on your decision to advance your career and obtain your Certified Case Manager (CCM) credential. Not long ago, I was in your shoes preparing to take the CCM Exam. I was disappointed when I found many of the books available were written by test prep companies with no input from case managers who had actually taken the exam. That may be why they were confusing and did not address many of the items CCMC stated would be on the exam.

I was looking for a concise resource without filler or fluff, just facts. But that book was not available. So I spent hundreds of hours reading books, in study groups, attending conferences and lectures, and searching the web. I took the information I found to help me pass the CCM and compiled it into an easy-to-read, comprehensive yet concise resource for you. The good news is you don't have to spend countless hours researching as I did. You have all the information you need right here!

Since the 1st edition was published in 2014, CCM Certification Made Easy has helped thousands of case managers pass the CCM Exam. It is now the most trusted resource for CCM Exam preparation. With each update of the exam, we update the book to make sure you have the most current information available.

Many updates have been made to this 3rd edition. First and most importantly, it was updated to the most recent exam blueprint. Secondly, at the request of our fans, practice questions were added. I also added a new first chapter to answer many of the questions we get and to help you get off to a great start. A little preparation goes a long way, so don't skip the first chapter!

In addition, I have many resources to help you pass that are not suitable for this book. I have added these as bonus material, and they can be found on the book website. The book has always included links to additional resources for you to continue your studies at the end of each chapter. To make it easier for you to access, these links are now on the book website so you can just click and go! I also broke up Chapter 2 into Parts 1 and 2 to make it easier for you to consume.

While making these improvements, I kept what everyone loved from the first 2 editions. Chapters 2-7 are titled the knowledge domains. Each chapter then addresses each subdomain addressed under that knowledge domain. These subdomains are **<u>bold with an underline</u>** for easy identification.

You will notice that we use the word "client" most of the time when referring to the person we are caring for. When working in an acute care setting we are used to referring to this person as the patient. In the insurance setting, this person is known as a member. While you may see both of these terms used in this book, we prefer to use the term client.

The term "patient" implies someone who is ill or injured and needs to be taken care of. Psychologically it puts us in a position of power while disempowering them. The term client implies that we are working for and with them, which we are.

And finally, to avoid using he/she all of the time, we have chosen to be consistent in using he for the client/patient/member, and she for the case manager. We understand that there are male and non-binary nurses and case managers. This decision was made solely for ease of reading and clarity between the case manager and patient.

Access Your FREE Bonus Material

To receive access to all of your FREE bonus material, go to the book website:

CCMcertificationMadeEasy.com

There, you will be able to access all of the bonus material including:

- Test Taking Strategies ($49 value)

- Free Companion Workbook ($10 value)

- 7 Day Mini-Course on creating your personal study plan ($29 value)

- Links to additional resources for each chapter

- Much more!

To access these resources, you will need to enter your email address and receipt number. If you purchased your book directly from us, you will receive an email with the number to enter. If you purchased from Amazon, the seller must be listed as Amazon. (Purchases from 3rd party sellers are not eligible for the bonus material.)

*Please note that to get the bonuses for free you must be the original purchaser of this book.

They are available for purchase for those who are not the original purchaser.

Upgrade your CCM certification journey with the

CCM Certification Made Easy App!

Get the ultimate study companion for your Android or iOS device —
the CCM Certification Made Easy App. Access interactive features,
practice exams, and valuable resources on the go, all in one place!

As a token of our appreciation for your book purchase,
we're excited to offer you an exclusive 30% discount on the
CCM Certification Made Easy App!

Simply scan the QR code below to claim this exclusive deal.

Unleash the full potential of your CCM preparation by combining the
book's comprehensive content with the interactive features of the app.
Don't miss out on this incredible opportunity to optimize your success!

Chapter One:
Getting Started

I know you are ready to begin studying the information but in my years of experience helping thousands of Case Managers obtain their CCM Certification, I have learned that to be successful in passing this test, you need to do more than just read the information. You have to understand the information as it aligns with CCMC's Philosophy of Case Management and CMSA's Standards of Practice for Case Managers.

In this first chapter, I will prepare you to study the material so that you understand it. But first, we will:

- Make sure you are eligible to sit for the exam,
- Learn about the application process, and
- Get to know the test.

By the end of this chapter, you will have the information you need to be knowledgeable and confident with your study plan and ultimately your test.

<<<< >>>>

About the Test

By passing this test and becoming a Certified Case Manager (CCM), you are joining an elite group of people. Not everyone can become a Certified Case Manager. There are eligibility requirements and an application process to sit for the exam, which after passing earns you the designation of board-certified case manager (CCM). The application process and exam ensure that case managers who hold the designation of CCM are of good moral character consistent with the CCMC Code of Professional Conduct, meet acceptable standards of quality in their practice, and possess an acceptable minimum level of basic knowledge with regard to the case management process.

Eligibility

You must meet the criteria in three categories to be eligible to sit for the CCM Exam; licensure or education, employment experience, and moral character. You must select the License/Certification option if you have a current, active, and unrestricted license or certification in a health or human services discipline that, within its scope of practice, allows you to conduct an assessment independently. It is important to note that the license must be active through the last date of the test administration that you are applying for.

If licensure or certification is not required for your discipline, you can apply with your degree. To be eligible to sit for the exam using your degree, you must have earned a baccalaureate or graduate degree in a health or human services field that promotes the physical, psychosocial, and/or vocational wellbeing of the persons being served. The degree must be from an institution that is fully accredited by a nationally recognized educational accreditation organization, and the individual must have completed a supervised field experience in case management, health, or behavioral health.

Information used with permission from the Commission for Case Manager Certification®. All rights reserved.

In addition to the licensure or education requirements, candidates for the CCM Exam must also satisfy employment experience requirements. This requirement must be satisfied at the time the application is submitted, not when the applicant will be testing. The applicant must have met one of the three employment criteria listed below.

1. 12 months of acceptable full-time case management employment experience supervised by a CCM who has been certified for at least 12 months.
2. 24 months of acceptable full-time case management employment experience.
3. 12 months of acceptable full-time case management employment experience as a supervisor of individuals who provide case management services.

Acceptable employment experience MUST meet all of the following conditions:

1. At least 20% of qualified work time must focus primarily on case management practice.
2. Perform at least four of The Five Core Components of Case Management which are:
   - Care Delivery and Reimbursement Methods
   - Psychosocial Concepts and Support Systems
   - Quality and Outcomes Evaluation and Measurements
   - Rehabilitation Concepts and Strategies
   - Ethical, Legal, and Practice Standards
3. Qualifying case management experience MUST be obtained in the United States, Puerto Rico, or the US Territories.

In addition, regarding number two above, within each of the core components performed, you must:

- Perform all Eight Essential Activities with Direct Client Contact; assessment, planning, implementation, coordination, monitoring, evaluation, outcomes, and general case management activities.

- Provide services across a continuum of care, beyond a single episode of care that addresses the ongoing needs of the individual being served.
- Be responsible for interacting with other relevant parties within the client's healthcare system.

All employment experience obtained within the past five years may be considered. Part-time employment experience will be prorated based on a 37-hour full-time workweek. Internship, preceptor-ship, practicum, and volunteer activities are NOT acceptable employment experience.

It is important to note that CCMC holds the applicant responsible for obtaining correct contact information for their supervisor(s). To expedite the application process I recommend that you contact the supervisor(s) in advance and notify them that they may receive a verification request.

The final criteria that must be met is moral character. You will be asked the following 8 questions:

1. Have you ever held a professional license or certification that was revoked, suspended, voluntarily relinquished, or placed on probation or otherwise been disciplined by a professional licensure or certification body?

2. Have you ever been reprimanded or discharged by an employer or supervisor for dishonesty in connection with your employment or occupation?

3. Have you ever been convicted of a felony?

4. During the last seven years, have you been arrested, accused, or convicted of violating any law or ordinance (excluding minor traffic violations)?

5. Have you ever been convicted of violating any law or ordinance dealing with the use, possession, or sale of drugs or alcohol?

6. Have you ever been convicted of violating any statute or ordinance dealing with sexual assault, abuse, molestation, indecent solicitation, obscenity, or similar acts of moral turpitude?

7. Have you ever received or been offered a grant of immunity in a grand jury proceeding?

8. Have you ever held yourself out to be a Certified Case Manager or used the initials CCM in the execution of any documents?

Additional information regarding eligibility can be found in CCMC's Certification Guide which can be downloaded from their website. After reviewing the Certification Guide, any remaining questions regarding eligibility should be directed to The Commission for Case Management Certification. Contact information can be found on their website CCMCertification.org. This is also where you will go to apply for the exam.

Eligibility Self-check
I meet the eligibility criteria because:

1. License/Certification or Education (Only a or b)

a. ☐ I have a license or certification that meets the criteria

    License/Certification type (RN, PT,etc.) _____

    License/Certification expiration date _____

    The license/certification will be valid through the testing month (Y/N) _____

b. ☐ I have a degree that meets the eligibility requirements

2. Employment Experience (only 1 is needed)

I have:

☐ 12 months of acceptable full-time case management employment experience supervised by a CCM who has been certified for at least 12 months.

☐ 24 months of acceptable full-time case management employment experience.

☐ 12 months of acceptable full-time case management employment experience as a supervisor of individuals who provide case management services.

    Supervisor's name: _____

    Supervisor's contact email: _____

3. ☐ I meet the moral character requirement.

Application Window

The CCM exam is given three times a year in April, August, and December. Candidates will be able to schedule the exam at any time during the test month based on availability at the testing center.

The application window to apply for the exam begins and ends several months before the exam month. At the time of publication, the exam cycle is as follows (check CCMCertification.org for the most up to date information)

Exam Cycle	August	December	April
Application window opens	March 1	July 1	November 1
Application window closes	May 31	September 30	January 31
Approval/ Denial Notification	By June 30	By October 31	By February 28
Exam administration	August 1-31	December 1-31	April 1-30

The Exam

The CCM exam consists of 180 multiple-choice questions. Of the 180 questions on the exam, only 150 are actual test questions that will be scored. The other 30 are pretest questions and are not used in the scoring of your exam. You will have three hours to complete the exam.

The content of the exam is based on an ongoing, nationwide validation research project. The research has identified five major domains of essential knowledge. Additionally, each of the five domains is further defined into sub-domains. The five domains and the number of questions for each domain are as follows:

- Care Delivery and Reimbursement Methods (28%) 40-44 questions
- Psychosocial Concepts and Support Systems (25%) 36-40 questions
- Quality and Outcomes Evaluation and Measurements (19%) 27-31 questions
- Rehabilitation Concepts and Strategies (11%) 14-18 questions
- Ethical, Legal, and Practice Standards (17%) 23-27 questions

This book is based on the above domains, with each chapter representing a domain. Within each chapter, each of the subdomains of that domain is addressed. You can find a complete list of the domains and subdomains by reviewing the table of contents as well as in the Certification Guide to the CCM Examination found at CCMCertification.org.

It is important to note that the content of the exam remains constant for each administration of the exam, but the actual questions will vary to protect the integrity of the examination process. Additionally, every five years the content of the exam (i.e. domains and subdomains) are reviewed, and updates are made to keep it up to date with the current practice of case management. The most recent update was for the December 2020 exam.

Information used with permission from the Commission for Case Manager Certification®. All rights reserved.

At the completion of the exam, candidates are provided an immediate pass/fail notification on the computer screen. This score is considered 99% accurate. Individuals who pass the exam are not to use the CCM credential until they receive their official CCM Certificate via mail (not the one printed at the testing center).

Setting Yourself Up For Success

Much of the following information is covered in greater detail in my free 7-day email mini-course that walks you through step-by-step how to create a personalized study plan based on your learning style and time until your test date. In this free mini-course, each day you will receive an email with information and an assignment to get you started with confidence on your journey to certification. There are also bonus videos and a special Facebook group just for this mini-course. For more information and to sign up for this FREE mini-course check out this book's resource page at CCMcertificationMadeEasy.com.

As stated previously, passing this test is not about memorizing facts. Instead, you must understand the information as it aligns with CCMC's Philosophy of Case Management and CMSA's Standards of Practice for Case Managers. In addition, you will need to understand how the information aligns with CCMC's Code of Professional Conduct for Case Managers and be familiar with their Glossary of Terms.

Before you begin studying, you need to understand the foundation the information will be built upon. For this reason, I highly recommend you start by reviewing the list of documents that follows. Once you have the foundation, you can begin building your knowledge on that foundation.

- CCMC Definition and Philosophy of Case Management
- CCMC Code of Professional Conduct for Case Managers

• CCMC Glossary of Terms

• CMSA Standards of Practice for Case Managers

The above resources (except for the Glossary of Terms) can be found in the appendix of this book. The Glossary of Terms can be printed, or the app can be purchased for your phone, making it easy to study from anywhere. When reviewing these documents for the first time, have multiple highlighters available. Information you know can be highlighted in one color (green) and the information you need to learn can be highlighted in another (pink). This will give you a good "at a glance" view of where you are starting from. All of that green will build your confidence, while the pink will help you easily identify the areas you need to work on.

Next review the knowledge domains and subdomains that you will be tested on. These can be found by reviewing the table of contents of this book, starting with Chapter 2. These can also be found in the Certification Guide to the CCM Examination at CCMCertification.org. Make sure to review the information for the date you are taking the test as the current guide has information for the test in August of 2020 as well as the test starting in December of 2020. I recommend using the two different colored highlighters for this also.

Once you have determined where your strengths and weaknesses lie, you will be able to determine how much information you need to learn. This, along with the amount of time you have until your exam date, will give you an idea of how much time you will need to devote to studying each week. I highly recommend that you schedule all of your study time now. Take out a calendar and schedule each week when you will study from now until your test date.

How To Use This Book To Pass Your Exam

This book was created with one purpose: to help you prepare for the CCM exam administered by the Commission for Case Management Certification.

It has been organized according to their most recent exam outline. Each chapter is a knowledge domain (with the exception of Chapters 2 and 3 which are parts 1 and 2 of the same knowledge domain).

Each chapter then addresses each subdomain addressed under that knowledge domain. These subdomains are **<u>bold with an underline</u>** for easy identification.

We have a Free Companion Workbook available that follows along with the book. In the workbook, key words and phrases are replaced with a blank line. While reading the book and following along in the workbook you can write in the words and phrases. This is helpful to those who learn best by writing. Go to CCMcertificationMadeEasy.com to download your Companion Workbook. (Please note that to get the Companion Workbook for free you must be the original purchaser of this book. It is available for purchase for those who are not the original purchaser.)

At the end of each chapter, you will find a mini test to test your knowledge of the information you just learned (this is after Chapter 3 for Chapters 2 and 3). In the appendix of this book, you will find a longer practice exam. Please remember that although these questions are very similar to what you will find on the exam, CCMC does not divulge the actual test questions. Any questions that may appear to be the same on the exam are purely coincidental.

Our goal with this book was to provide a concise, yet comprehensive resource for you to use to prepare for the exam. But there may be areas you want to research further. To assist you with this we have added references at the end of each chapter. In addition, we have a list of online references where you can find additional, trustworthy information. Because the website URLs are often long and confusing, we have provided the links on our website so that you can just click and go! These can be found at CCMcertificationMadeEasy.com.

Additional Resources

You will find numerous free resources on the website dedicated to this book, CCMcertificationMadeEasy.com to help you pass the exam. In addition, to help you grow in the profession we have a Facebook group with over 14,000 casemanagers that I would like to personally invite you to join. There you will find and provide information, support, and encouragement in a friendly environment of peers.

And finally, if you are someone who learns best by hearing the information or needs accountability to stay motivated, we have additional resources for you. We offer two CCM Prep Courses. The first is On-Demand and available anytime from anywhere with an internet connection. The course is self-paced and can be viewed over and over. It is best for someone who needs repetition, to hear the information, or both.

The second is an Online Live 6-Week Course. The Online Live Course is offered three times a year, corresponding with each testing cycle. The classes are held 2 hours a week for 6 weeks and taught by two live instructors. You have access to your instructors during the class and between classes via email. Before each class, there is required reading from this book. This is best for someone who needs to hear the information but also wants accountability, motivation, and interaction with an instructor. More information on our course offerings is available on our website, CCMcertificationMadeEasy.com.

Chapter Two:
Care Delivery and
Reimbursement Methods
Part 1

Care Delivery and Reimbursement Methods comprises 28% of the exam with between 40 and 44 questions on this topic. It is the largest area of the exam. This has been divided into two parts for easier reading.

****

This chapter will introduce the case management process, roles and functions of case management, as well as other foundational material related to the practice of case management. As case managers, we often do without understanding the why behind it. This chapter will help you begin to understand why we do what we do.

<<<< >>>>

Collaborative/Comprehensive/Integrated/Holistic Case Management Services

Both the Commission for Case Management Certification (CCMC) and the Case Management Society of America (CMSA) address in their philosophies of case management the collaborative, comprehensive, integrative, and holistic approach that must be present in case management. The very definition of case management states that it is a collaborative process.

The Commission for Case Manager Certification (CCMC) defines case management as "a collaborative process that assesses, plans, implements, coordinates, monitors, and evaluates the options and services required to meet the client's health and human services needs. It is characterized by advocacy, communication, and resource management and promotes quality and cost-effective interventions and outcomes."

In their Philosophy and Guiding Principles, they state that case managers approach the delivery of case-managed health and human services in a collaborative manner. Professionals from within or across healthcare organizations (e.g., provider, employer, payer, and community agencies) and work settings work together closely for the benefit of clients/support systems.

They go on to state that the case management process is holistic in that it addresses the medical, physical, emotional, financial, psychosocial, behavioral, and other needs of the client as well as their support system. The goals of case management are first and foremost focused on improving clients' clinical, functional, emotional, and psychosocial status.

Based on the cultural beliefs, values, and needs of the clients/support systems, and in collaboration with all service providers (both healthcare professionals and paraprofessionals), case managers link clients/support systems with appropriate providers of care and resources throughout the continuum of health and human services and across various care settings. They do so while ensuring that the care provided is safe, effective, client-centered, timely, efficient, and equitable.

CMSA's Standards of Practice 2016 state in their Statement of Philosophy that, "The key philosophical components of case management address care that is holistic and client-centered, with mutual goals, allowing stewardship of resources for the client and the health care system including the diverse group of stakeholders. Through these efforts, case management focuses simultaneously on achieving optimal health and attaining wellness to the highest level possible for each client."

And later in their Guiding Principles, they state that case managers:

1. Use a client-centric, collaborative partnership approach that is responsive to the individual client's culture, preferences, needs, and values; and

2. Use a comprehensive, holistic, and compassionate approach to care delivery that integrates a client's medical, behavioral, social, psychological, functional, and other needs.

Integrated Case Management (ICM)

In addition to the integrative case management performed when linking clients with providers and resources throughout the continuum of care, there is another definition of integrated case management that must be mentioned.

Patients who have both medical and behavioral conditions have unique needs. Integrated Case Management (ICM) addresses both the physical and mental health of the client to enhance their health, wellness, level of functioning, and quality of life.

According to the National Comorbidity Survey, of individuals with a mental illness, 68% also have a physical health condition such as cardiovascular disease, diabetes, or hypertension. These high-need individuals often receive uncoordinated care that results in higher costs and poorer health outcomes.

People with mental illnesses and substance use disorders typically receive most of their care in community behavioral healthcare settings. Many are unable or unwilling to receive care in a primary care setting. Even when they do, coordination between behavioral health and medical services may be poor. For those individuals who have relationships with behavioral health organizations, care may be best delivered by bringing primary care, prevention services, and wellness activities onsite at behavioral health settings. This method is known as integrated healthcare.

Case Management Models, Process, and Tools

The Commission for Case Manager Certification (CCMC) defines case management as "a collaborative process that assesses, plans, implements, coordinates, monitors, and evaluates the options and services required to meet the client's health and human services needs. It is characterized by advocacy, communication, and resource management and promotes quality and cost-effective interventions and outcomes."

According to CCMC's Case Management Body of Knowledge, the case management process consists of:

- Screening
- Stratifying risk
- Assessing
- Planning
- Implementing (care coordination)
- Following-up
- Transitioning (transitional care)
- Communication post-transition
- Evaluation

These steps are not sequential, meaning case managers do not complete a phase and check it off their list as complete. Many phases will take place concurrently, or be revisited and repeated. For example, a new problem may arise during follow-up with a patient. The case manager would then return to the planning phase for that problem while continuing to follow up on the original problem.

Screening

Case management is not for every client. During the screening phase, patient information is reviewed to decide the patient's appropriateness for case management services. Details obtained may include claims information, utilization of healthcare services, current health status, insurance eligibility, support system, and health history.

Depending on the program, clients may be appropriate for case management based on:

- Diagnosis
- High-dollar diagnosis
- High utilization (frequent hospital or emergency room visits)
- Poor pain control
- Chronic, catastrophic illness
- Social issues, such as a weak or nonexistent support system
- Difficult discharge planning
- Financial issues

Stratifying Risk

Case managers use biometric screening and health risk assessment tools to classify clients into low, moderate, or high-risk categories. This allows for proper interventions based on the client's needs.

Risk stratification can also be done before screening to identify members who could benefit from case management. Many population management, chronic care management, and health insurance settings use technology to stratify risk and identify clients that may be most appropriate for their case management services. This technology may flag all cases with certain diagnoses, high-dollar claims, or frequent hospitalizations, for example.

Assessing

A comprehensive, needs-based assessment is conducted based on the case manager's practice setting to identify the client's problems, needs, and interests. The assessment can be done in-person or telephonically. In addition to speaking with the client, information can also be obtained from family, caregivers, providers, medical records, insurance representatives, the client's employer, and other sources. This information is then used to create a case management plan of care. The assessment phase is similar to screening but provides a more in-depth look at the client's healthcare situation. The assessment may include:

- Medical history
- Current medical conditions
- Functional status
- Cognitive status
- Health insurance status
- Spiritual life
- Psychosocial concerns
- Environment (e.g., living conditions)
- Vocational/educational status
- Financial status
- Support system

- Culture and language
- Self-care capability
- Health literacy
- Health goals
- Readiness to change
- Past and current service utilization
- Current medications
- Safety

Planning

The objective of this phase is to develop an individualized case management plan of care to address the identified needs. This should be done with input from the client and/or caregiver and other members of the healthcare team whenever possible. Short-term and long-term goals should be developed and prioritized, and interventions should be planned. The short-term goals should be directly related to the long-term goals. The interventions are the treatments, resources, and services needed to meet the client's needs and goals and should apply evidence-based standards and care guidelines. The acronym SMART is used to identify the attributes of effective goals.

- **S**pecific
- **M**easurable
- **A**chievable
- **R**ealistic
- **T**ime-bound

The planning phase is completed after services, treatments, and resources needed are identified and authorizations are obtained from the payer.

Implementing

The case management plan is carried out during the implementation phase, also called care coordination. The interventions arranged in the planning phase are executed, coordinated, and secured. The case manager acts as a liaison between the client, caregivers, providers, and payers.

Following-Up/Monitoring

The case manager conducts ongoing assessments and gathers information from the patient, caregiver, and other relevant sources. This information is evaluated to determine the client's response to the current case management plan and the progress toward the desired outcomes. Modifications are made to the plan as needed, and ongoing follow-ups determine the effectiveness of the modifications.

Transitional Care

Transitions of care, whether across the health and human services continuum, to differing levels of care, to another case manager, or from the case management program, put the client at increased risk for adverse events. Case managers provide a valuable service by overseeing the proper transition to the next level of care, as well as ensuring continuity of care.

During this phase, the case manager prepares the client for discharge or transfer to another provider. She coordinates communication among the client, the current provider, the subsequent provider, and caregivers.

**See subdomain-section on Transitions of Care/Transitional Care.

Post-transition Communication

After a client transitions from an episode of care, the case manager contacts the client and/or caregiver to confirm a smooth transition. The case manager ensures post-transition services are being obtained, reconciles medications, and assesses for issues.

Evaluating Outcomes

The case manager assesses the effectiveness of the case management plan of care, its effect on the client's condition, and creates any associated reports.

The evaluation may focus on multiple aspects of care, including:

- A financial evaluation with a cost-benefit analysis and return on investment
- Clinical outcomes
- Quality of life
- Client satisfaction
- Self-care management ability
- Knowledge of health conditions and plan of care

Case Management Models

There are numerous Case Management Models used today. All models focus on the following three roles:

(1) Patient-flow, making sure the patient moves through the acute care setting in a timely manner;

(2) Utilization Management (UM) - communicating with payer sources;

(3) Discharge Planning (DCP) - Moving the patient to the next level of care. This includes assessing the needs the patient may have after they leave the acute care setting and ensuring the safe, timely, and appropriate discharge with the resources needed.

Who carries out the role is what differentiates each model. Most case management models are a variation of one of the following:

Integrated CM Model - All roles; patient flow, UM, and DCP, are performed by a single nurse case manager. In this model, a Social Worker may be consulted when appropriate.

Dyad model - RN and SW CMs work together in one department. They may co-manage the patient; where the RN deals with education and clinical issues, and the SW focuses on financial, social, and discharge needs. Alternatively, an initial assessment may be performed and after determining the primary needs of the client (medical vs social) one would take on the responsibility of the client with the other available as a resource.

Triad model / Collaborative Case Management (UM/CM/SW) - This model is similar to the Dyad Model, but a third person is involved who takes over the Utilization Manager (UM) activities working with the third-party payers, leaving the RN and SW CMs to focus on patient flow, transitions, and DCP.

There are strengths and weaknesses to all of these models for example…

With the integrated model, the case manager really knows the case. She is in direct communication with the patient, payer, vendors, physicians, and other staff. This reduces duplication and fragmentation which may be more cost and time-efficient. On the other hand, it is more time consuming and requires adequate staffing.

The Collaborative Model eliminates the very time-consuming UM task for the case manager. This allows the case manager to focus on other functions. It does, though, require great communication between the team members and works best if all team members are in the same department and report to the same supervisor. There can also be some redundancy with this model, such as assessments and chart review.

Roles and Functions of Case Managers in Various Care/ Practice Settings

Many case management roles and functions are the same regardless of setting, such as advocacy, assessment, planning, empowerment, facilitation, collaboration, and education. For example, all case managers conduct comprehensive assessments of the client's needs. From the assessment, the case manager develops a case management plan in collaboration with the patient and family.

Case managers also collaborate with the client and his family, caregiver, physician, provider, payer, and community to achieve quality, cost-efficient outcomes. This requires the case manager to facilitate communication and coordination between all members involved in the patient's care. She must also educate the client, family, and members of the healthcare team regarding treatment options, insurance benefits, and community resources to facilitate informed decision-making. This empowers the client and promotes self-advocacy.

Advocacy for both the client and the payer is another role of the case manager. The goal is to achieve the best outcome for the client, provider, and payer. If a conflict arises, the client's needs take priority.

The setting the case manager works in often determines the extent to which each of these functions is carried out. Furthermore, unique roles and functions may exist in a particular case management setting. Below is a list of settings in which case managers practice, followed by functions of case managers in those settings.

1. Physician's offices, ambulatory care clinics, accountable care organizations, corporations, and community-based organizations, including healthcare centers and university clinics. These roles are geared toward prevention.
   - Wellness programs
   - Screenings
   - Health risk assessments
   - Risk-reduction strategies
   - Telephonic triage

- Disease management
- Facilitating access to services
- Referrals to community-based resources
- Coordination of medical and social services
- Ensuring patient knowledge and compliance with treatment
- Monitoring

2. Hospitals
   - Utilization review
   - Discharge planning
   - Resource management
   - Coordination of care among team members
   - Transition to post-acute care

3. Acute inpatient rehabilitation, subacute care, long term acute care hospitals (LTAC), and skilled nursing facilities (SNF)
   - Coordinate interdisciplinary team (IDT) meetings
   - Verify benefits and authorization of services
   - Facilitate referrals
   - Discharge planning

4. Payer-based settings, including public health insurance programs (Medicare, Medicaid, state-funded programs) and private health insurance programs (occupational health, disability, group health insurance, managed care organizations)
   - Liaise between providers, members, and insurance company
   - Coordinate care
   - Ensure appropriate care
   - Negotiate for services

- Monitor for compliance with treatment plan
- Ensure appropriate level of care and care setting
- Educate on healthcare benefits
- Utilization management
- Discharge planning

5. Palliative care, home care, and hospice care

Case managers in these settings combine the role of caregiver with case manager. The case manager may have hands-on nursing responsibilities.

- Liaise with providers
- Communicate with treating physicians
- Provide patient and family education
- Assess for and coordinate additional services and durable medical equipment (DME)
- Provide skilled nursing care

6. Workers' compensation organizations

Case management in workers' compensation cases focuses on vocational activities, such as collaborating with the employer to get the employee back to work.

- Facilitate communication between the employer, claims adjuster, union representative, state administrative agency, attorneys and providers
- Coordinate care between multiple healthcare providers
- Monitor progress
- Utilization review
- Obtain precertification when necessary
- Perform job analysis
- Accompany injured workers during physician appointments

In addition, there are subspecialties of case management that have very unique roles and functions such as Vocational Case Managers who assist employees to return to work as quickly as possible.

Life care planning is a subspecialty of case management and other professions. It provides a comprehensive care plan for the health needs of an individual who has experienced a catastrophic injury or has chronic healthcare needs. A life care planner completes a comprehensive assessment, data analysis, and research to provide an organized and concise plan for the present and future needs of an individual. Life care plans are used by:

- Attorneys, to determine future care cost for a client
- Treatment teams, to provide a plan for ongoing treatment and follow up
- Trust managers, to identify scheduled needs and associated costs
- Patients and families, to coordinate and facilitate resources

Caseload Considerations

Many factors determine the caseload capacity of a case manager. A case manager who conducts face-to-face case management in a rural area cannot manage the same caseload as a telephonic case manager, due to logistical and transportation factors. And complex cases require more time and involvement from the case manager than disease management cases, for example.

Because of the multiple factors and complexity of determining an appropriate caseload, the Case Management Society of America (CMSA) created a Case Load Capacity Calculator tool (http://clcc.cm-innovators.com/). This online tool* was open for public use after registering. It took into account several factors to determine the appropriate caseload for a case manager.

Please note that this tool has been deactivated, pending update and revision.

These factors include:

- Profession (nurse/social worker)
- Setting (clinic, hospital, subacute, health plan, workers' compensation)
- Other roles the case manager performs (behavioral health, utilization management, disease management, supervisory roles, preceptor/trainer)
- Complexity of cases
- Experience of case manager
- Length of time in current role
- Site-based technology (hand-written reports, one information technology system, multiple information technology systems)
- Types of contact (face-to-face, telephonic)
- Non-case management activities (meetings, continuing education, travel, training)

In 2008, the Case Management Caseload Concept Paper, a joint effort of CMSA and the National Association of Social Workers (NASW) was released. This paper had a threefold goal of:

1. To compile a comprehensive list of elements that can impact potential caseload determinations in complex and diverse CM setting.

2. To organize these identified elements into a schematic matrix useful for preliminary evaluation of factors that impact caseloads.

3. To enhance professional CM practice, thereby promoting quality care outcomes for clients and patients.

The consensus arrived at by the CMSA/NASW Case Management Caseload Concept Paper (2008) was that the "higher the number of cases assigned at any given time, then the larger the number of responsibilities and greater frequency of encounters the case managers must accomplish to perform their roles adequately."

According to The Caseload Guidebook for Successful Outcomes (2013), the size of caseloads differs depending on the model in practice and practice setting. The practice setting also affects the potential number of patients/ clients/members that can be impacted as well. CMSA/NASW also identifies that the skill set and experience level of the individual case manager plays a large role in the number of clients that can be managed with higher acuity. Recommendations for acute care caseloads by the Center for Case Management (CCM) for acute care case managers (revised, 2013) were based on the case mix index, which is a determinant of potential patient case management acuity.

Several projects have been initiated over the years to look at caseload versus workload; volume versus acuity to ensure that a patient's needs and outcomes are maximized while at the same time maximizing the efficacy of the individual case manager. Acuity based concepts, "client-need severity; case management intervention severity and case management activity dose, have been utilized at different times (2001, 2006, 2009) to develop instruments such as, the CM Acuity Tool, the Acuity Tool, AccuDiff and automated acuity scoring systems which access the severity, intensity, and complexity of case management cases, with the aim of balancing caseload/workload to provide patients with the services and resources they need to have a safe discharge and successful post-intervention/hospitalization, decreasing case manager's stress and increasing productivity and efficacy.

Goals and Objectives of Case Management Practice

Goals and objectives of case management include:
- Achieving client goals
- Client autonomy
- Client knowledge of disease process, prognosis, and treatment options
- Optimum health and functioning for the client

- Client ability to self-advocate
- Informed decision-making by the client
- Appropriate use of services and resources
- Timeliness of services
- Quality of care
- Appropriate level of care to meet client needs
- Optimal level of client independence
- Achieving optimal outcomes

Negotiation Techniques

Managed care contracts have decreased the need for price negotiations between case managers and providers, as pricing is set in advance. Even so, negotiating cost is still required in some situations, such as when services are not covered by the managed care contract or when working with out-of-network providers. Case managers may negotiate for services, such as length of stay, approval of needed services, and extra-contractual benefits.

What is negotiation, and how can case managers use it effectively?

Negotiation is the reaching of an agreement through discussion and compromise. The aim of negotiation is to explore the situation and find a mutually acceptable solution. There are two types of negotiation: aggressive/hardball and cooperative.

Aggressive or hardball negotiation aims to result in a winner and a loser. Tactics include intimidation, manipulation, tricks, and ridicule. The aggressive negotiator makes few concessions but extreme demands. He or she may threaten to cease negotiations. This type of negotiation often fails to reach an agreement. It results in mistrust and damages future negotiations. It is not recommended for case managers, as it can result in deadlock, leaving the patient without needed services.

Cooperative negotiation seeks a win-win outcome and usually results in the best end for everyone. The negotiator is trustworthy, objective, fair, and reasonable.

This approach results in agreements faster and more often than the aggressive technique and facilitates future negotiations.

The Negotiation Process

The key to the negotiation process is being prepared, developing a relationship with the other party, and establishing a common ground in the best interest of the client. Showing respect for the other party can be as simple as returning a voicemail or email promptly. Respect builds trust, which will enhance the negotiation process.

Communication is as important as respect in the negotiation process. It includes not only what you say, but also how you say it and how well you listen. In face-to-face communication, it also includes body language. Be clear and concise, and engage in active listening by paying attention (rather than planning how you will respond). Summarize the other person's comments and ask questions to clarify and ensure you understand his points.

Negotiation starts with preparation, so conduct research to understand the other person's side before meeting. (If negotiating price, know competitors' pricing.) Next, establish the problems and the goals with the other party. Failure to agree upon goals can make the negotiation process difficult.

Once the goals are established, determine what areas you agree on—these can be put aside—and what areas you disagree on. On the areas where there is disagreement, begin to work toward compromise. The negotiation is deemed successful when a mutually acceptable resolution is obtained.

The case manager can use negotiation effectively with patients, caregivers, and physicians, as well as payers and vendors. Once relationships are built, subsequent negotiations will be smoother and more enjoyable.

Case managers use negotiation to:
- Develop a realistic plan of care with patients and care providers
- Obtain approval for needed services
- Control cost
- Obtain benefits outside of the benefit contract
- Determine length of stay

Physical Functioning and Behavioral Health Assessment

The Activities of Daily Living (ADLs) and the more advanced Instrumental Activities of Daily Living (IADLs) are assessment tools that evaluate areas of essential function for self-care and independence.

ADLs measure the level of independence on performing six basic activities:
- Bathing
- Dressing
- Toileting/continence
- Transferring
- Hygiene/grooming
- Feeding

The ADLs can be easily remembered by the mnemonic DEATH: Dressing/ bathing, Eating, Ambulating, Toileting, Hygiene.

The IADLs tool assesses the ability to perform eight independent living skills that are more complex than the basic ADLs assessment. These include:
- Shopping
- Using the telephone
- Paying bills/budgeting
- Food preparation
- Housekeeping

- Laundry
- Using transportation
- Handling medications

The Patient Health Questionnaire-2 (PHQ-2) pre-screens for depression. Clients who pre-screen positive for depression should be evaluated further with the Patient Health Questionnaire-9 (PHQ-9), which is the most common screening tool to identify depression. It asks the patient to rate the frequency of nine problems occurring over the previous two weeks on a scale ranging from 0 (not at all) to 3 (nearly every day), including little interest or pleasure in doing things, and feeling down, depressed, or hopeless.

Differences in and Application of Age-Specific Care

Each age group has unique characteristics and needs:
- Physical, including motor/sensory attributes
- Psychosocial and developmental tasks
- Cognitive and intellectual functioning
- Major fears and stressors

Accreditation bodies, such as The Joint Commission (TJC) and URAC, require organizations to define the client population it serves, and the age groups within that client population. The organization is then charged with assessing the competence of staff to address the special needs and behaviors of the specific age groups it serves.

Many organizations define the following four categories:
- Neonatal and infant
- Child and adolescent
- Adult
- Geriatric

However, some facilities identify additional subcategories depending upon the population served.

Case managers need to be able to assess, communicate with, and create a case management plan of care for the client population they serve in a way that is appropriate with the client's age and capabilities.

Case managers apply age-specific considerations when:
- Performing physical assessment and interpreting the findings
- Assessing and addressing nutritional status
- Communicating
- Involving the client in care and decision making
- Providing instruction and education
- Selecting medical equipment and supplies
- Assisting the patient to cope
- Assessing risk for injury and instituting preventive measures

When assessing the client, it is important to use specialized assessment tools appropriate for the client's age. Examples include pediatric pain assessment tools, cognitive assessment tools for elders, and fall risk assessment tools. Refer to the policies and procedures your organization has created to guide the use of specific tools.

As you manage patients in different age groups, keep in mind that there are specific psychological and physiological needs. These vary by age group or by developmental level. By understanding these differences, you can provide more individualized care to your patients. We will review these in the next section.

Life Span Considerations

We will now look at age-specific groups throughout the lifespan including Erikson's stage of psychosocial development, risk prevention, and other notable considerations for each age group. There may be slight variations in the way groups are organized depending on the source referenced or a slight overlapping as changes do not occur immediately when the age is reached.

Age-specific Groups at a Glance

- Neonates: 1 day to 28 days
- Infants: 29 days to 1 year
- Toddlers: 1 year to 3 years
- Child: 3-12
    - Preschool: 3 years to 5 years
    - School-aged: 6 years to 12 years
- Adolescent: 13 years to 18 years
    - Young adolescents:13 years to15 years
    - Older adolescents: 16 years to 18 years
- Adult: 19 years to 65 years
    - Young adult: 19 years to 40 years
    - Middle-aged adult: ages 40 years to 65 years
- Elder: 65 years and older
    - Young old: 65 years to 75 years
    - Old: 75 years to 85 years
    - Old old: 85 years and older

Neonates: ages 1 day to 28 days

Developmental Task: Trust versus Mistrust, development of the ability to rely on others.

Risk assessment and teaching related to:

- Sudden Infant Death Syndrome (SIDS) preventive interventions
- Risk for both hypothermia and hyperthermia due to immature heat regulation system

- Risk for dehydration due to immature renal function, high metabolic rate, and insensible fluid loss
- Risk for infection due to an immature immune system

Infants: ages 29 days to 1 year

Developmental Task: Trust versus Mistrust, development of the ability to rely on others.

Risk assessment and teaching related to:

- Accident prevention: Curiosity, energy, impulsiveness, and lack of inhibition lead to unsafe situations.
- Choking prevention: The infant is in Freud's oral stage of development and often will put things in their mouth.
- Immunizations

Other Considerations: Infants learn to play, but play alone rather than engaging with other children.

Toddlers: ages 1 year to 3 years

Developmental Task: Autonomy versus Shame or Doubt, focused on developing a sense of personal control over physical skills and a sense of independence.

Risk assessment and teaching related to:

- Accident prevention: Curiosity, energy, impulsiveness, and lack of inhibition lead to unsafe situations.
- Immunizations

Other Considerations:

- Toilet training is a major developmental task for this age group.
- Toddlers have a short attention span.
- Toddlers learn to walk and talk during this stage.

Child: ages 3 years to 12 years

We will further divide this age group into two subcategories: preschool and school-aged.

Preschool: ages 3 years to 5 years

Developmental Task: Initiative versus guilt, focused on exploring and seeking answers. The preschooler feels guilty if they make a mistake or disappoints parents.

Risk assessment and teaching related to:

- High risk for accidental injury
- Immunizations

Other Considerations:

- Likes to play with others and may have imaginary friends

School-aged: 6 years to 12 years

Developmental Task: Industry versus Inferiority. The school-aged child desires to make things, solve problems, and master tasks. Doing so builds feelings of confidence and prevents the feeling of inadequacy.

Risk assessment and teaching related to:

- Safety
- Immunizations
- Nutrition habits

Other Considerations:

- School-age children begin to compare themselves with others.

Adolescent: ages 13 years to 18 years

Developmental Task: Identity Formation versus Identity Confusion. Adolescents search for a sense of self and personal identity through an intense exploration of personal values, beliefs, and goals. This may include separating from parents and authority figures and developing relationships with the opposite sex.

Risk assessment and teaching related to:

- Seek follow-up referral or resources if you identify indications of depression or suicidal thoughts. Suicide is the third most frequent cause of death in this age group
- Assess nutritional needs due to growth spurts
- For females, teaching related to menarche
- Acne
- Illicit substance use and sexual activity

Other Considerations:

- Adolescents are particularly concerned about body image and appearing different from their peers.
- Hormonal changes can make adolescents emotionally labile.
- May think they are invincible and may engage in high-risk behaviors.

This group can be subdivided into two groups:

- Young adolescents, ages 13 years to 15 years
- Older adolescents, ages 16 years to 18 years

Adult: 19 years to 65 years

We will further divide this age group into two subcategories: young adult and middle-aged adult.

Young adult: ages 20 years to 40 years

Developmental Task: Intimacy versus Self-isolation. Reaching out, and forming an intimate, loving, and committed relationship with another person.

Risk assessment and teaching related to:

- Regular check-ups
- Update immunizations (tetanus, hepatitis, flu)
- Promote a healthy lifestyle (nutrition, exercise)
- Inform about health risks (heart disease, diabetes, cancer)
- Stress reduction

Other Considerations:

- With consent, involve significant other or other support systems.
- Career and interpersonal goals are important to the young adult.
- May have many responsibilities including work, relationship with significant other, and raising children.

Middle-aged adults: ages 40 years to 65 years

Developmental Task: Generativity versus Self-absorption. Generativity refers to "leaving a legacy" by contributing to the next generation and to society. The concern about providing for others is equal to the concern about providing for self.

Risk assessment and teaching related to:

- For females, teaching related to menopause
- Screening tests such as mammograms, bone density, and PSA
- Development of chronic disease
- Encourage regular check-ups and preventive care

Other Considerations:

- Middle-aged adults are at the peak of their influence and authority.
- Forced dependency in the patient role can be distressing.
- Many are caring for children and aging parents (sandwich generation).
- With consent, involve a spouse or significant other.

Elder: 65 years and older

Developmental Task: Ego Integrity versus Despair. The contemplation of accomplishments and the acceptance of the life lived.

Risk assessment and teaching related to:

- Increased risk for dehydration
- Increased sensitivity to medications (dosages may need to be adjusted)
- Alteration in senses such as vision and hearing as well as balance can put at an increased risk for falls
- Increased incidence of cancer
- Skin becomes thin and frail

Other Considerations:

- This age group is faced with many losses. The progressive loss of memory, physical capabilities, independence, spouse, peers.
- There can be a large difference in the health and needs of this category. Some will have failing health while others will remain healthy and active until death.

People are living longer. Many are delaying retirement or starting a second career later in life. This has resulted in the redefining of the term elderly. This group can be subdivided into three groups:

- Young old, ages 65 years to 75 years
- Old, ages 75 years to 85 years
- Old old, ages 85 years and older

Management of Clients with Acute and Chronic Illness(es)

Acute diseases are characterized by a rapid onset with a short duration. Appendicitis, flu, pneumonia, acute respiratory distress syndrome, and acute renal failure are examples of acute illnesses. In contrast, chronic diseases require a lifetime of management, such as diabetes, lupus, heart failure, and chronic renal failure.

An acute disease may lead to a chronic disease. Take, for example, a patient with acute onset of multisystem organ failure requiring a ventilator and dialysis.

If the patient is unable to wean from the ventilator or if kidney function does not return, the patient has developed a chronic condition.

In managing a patient with acute illness, the case manager should assess whether the patient will be able to return to his prior living arrangement. The case manager should also assess for any needs the patient may have upon discharge, such as home health care or durable medical equipment. If the patient is unable to return home directly from the hospital, the case manager facilitates transfer to inpatient rehabilitation, a long-term acute care hospital, or another suitable facility.

Patients with a chronic disease must be taught to manage their condition to prevent morbidities and comorbidities. This includes medication management, lifestyle and dietary changes, and testing and follow-up with their healthcare provider. They must be educated on the benefits of treatment and the risks of noncompliance. They must understand that chronic diseases will not be cured, but rather managed, so they have a better quality of life.

Acute and chronic illness(es) are disruptions to the patient's and family's lifestyle. Family members may have to take on additional responsibilities and rely on support systems. The case manager may make referrals to support groups or counselors, financial resources, or disease-based agencies.

Management of Clients with Disability(ies)

CCMC in their Glossary of Terms (2019) defines Disability Case Management as a process of managing occupational and nonoccupational disease with the aim of returning the disabled employee to a productive work schedule and employment. Occupational diseases are the result of an injury on the job or illness caused by the work environment. Nonoccupational diseases are health conditions that are not related to the work environment but result in short- or long-term disability that prevents the return to work. Examples can include but are not limited to traumatic brain injury, cancer, and motor vehicle accident.

To best manage these clients, the case manager needs to be well versed in both workers' compensation and rehabilitation concepts, strategies, benefits, and laws. Disability case managers support the long and short term financial, psychological, social, physical, sexual, and vocational needs of the disabled individual.

When the injury or illness occurs, the immediate focus is to limit the disability by coordinating and facilitating medical interventions and facilitating referrals to rehabilitation providers and specialists. The ultimate goal of care and services is to return the patient to work and to restore optimal level of functioning and independence as soon as possible.

Adherence to Care Regimen

Depending on the disease, it is estimated that 40-70% of patients do not adhere to their care regimen. Nonadherence means not carrying out the treatment plan or carrying it out incorrectly, and includes the failure to keep appointments, follow lifestyle changes, maintain dietary changes, and take medication as prescribed.

It is estimated that the cost of nonadherence is $100-300 billion annually. In addition to the financial implications, there are clinical implications, such as

decreased quality of life and premature death. An important task case managers perform is monitoring for and increasing patient adherence to care regimens.

Poor adherence to the care regimen leads to:

- Decreased quality of life
- Higher healthcare costs
- Increased emergency department visits
- Increased hospitalizations
- Avoidable nursing home admissions
- Decreased productivity
- Poor clinical outcomes
- Premature death

Conversely, improved patient adherence leads to better health outcomes, better chronic care management, improved population health, improved quality of life and productivity, and lower healthcare costs. Patient adherence is especially important for the long-term management of chronic diseases, such as kidney disease, heart disease, and diabetes.

There are numerous reasons for patient nonadherence, both intentional and unintentional. In some cases, the patient feels the care regimen is too bothersome, complex, or unnecessary. In other instances, there may be poor communication between the patient and the healthcare provider or poor health literacy leading to misunderstanding of the care regimen. It is also not uncommon for patients to forget portions of what they were told by the provider. The medical industry is becoming increasingly complex, often leading to complex treatment plans. The more complex the treatment plan, the less likely a patient will adhere to it.

The case manager can increase adherence to the care regimen in several ways. The first is to assess the client's knowledge and understanding of his condition and care regimen. A patient's adherence can be directly correlated to his understanding.

Next, the case manager should get to know the client and develop a trusting relationship with him. Especially when dealing with complex care regimens, client knowledge alone is not enough to increase adherence. Understanding the client's beliefs, attitudes, support system, and self-efficacy will help the case manager communicate with the client and foster collaboration.

Once the case manager has a better understanding of what the client needs to know and what will motivate the client to adhere to the care regimen, she can begin to educate the client. For effective education:

- Use simple language, avoiding medical jargon
- Limit instructions to 3-4 major points during each discussion
- Supplement teaching with written materials when appropriate
- Involve the client's family or caregiver
- Evaluate client understanding
- Reinforce concepts previously taught

For clients with complex care regimens, case managers can use the Health Belief Model to optimize behavior change and adherence by ensuring that clients:

- Perceive themselves to be at risk due to lack of adoption of healthy behavior (perceived susceptibility)
- Perceive their medical conditions to be serious (perceived severity)
- Believe in the positive effects of the suggested treatment (perceived benefits)
- Have channels to address their fears and concerns (perceived barriers)
- Perceive themselves as having the requisite skills to perform the health behavior (self-efficacy)

By understanding which of these beliefs is lacking, the case manager can tailor interventions to meet the needs of the client.

Medication Adherence

According to a 2018 article published by the National Institutes of Health, studies show that nonadherence to medications causes 125,000 deaths annually and accounts for 10-25% of hospital and nursing home admissions in the United States. Overall, nearly 75% of adults are nonadherent in one or more ways.

The consequences of medication nonadherence are vast. Not only does the patient fail to benefit from the effects of the medication, but when the prescribing physician assumes that the patient is taking the medication as prescribed, he or she may make inappropriate medication, dosage, or treatment plan changes, which can result in further complications or adverse health outcomes. Creating a new illness is also a risk; for example, antibiotic-resistant bacteria came about due to patients not completing their courses of antibiotics.

Nonadherence to medications takes many forms, including primary nonadherence, such as not filling the prescription, and secondary nonadherence, such as not taking the prescription as prescribed (e.g., changing the dosage or frequency, stopping before completing the course of therapy, filling the prescription but never taking the medication, skipping or missing doses, or not refilling the prescription).

Factors that negatively affect adherence include:
- Side effects
- High copays or costs
- No noticeable symptoms of the disease (for example, hypercholesterolemia and hypertension do not produce noticeable symptoms)
- Multiple doses per day

To increase medication adherence, the case manager should first understand why the client is nonadherent. For example, if side effects are a problem, the solution could be to take the medication with food or to change the time of day it is taken. The client or case manager should discuss with the prescribing physician the inability to take the medication. An alternative medication may be prescribed, or one that counteracts the side effects.

If the client often forgets to take his medication, alarms, text messages, medication boxes, apps, and other reminders may help, or he could associate it with something in his daily routine, such as eating breakfast, going to bed, or brushing his teeth.

Reducing the number of pills or the frequency they are taken can also increase adherence. The physician may be able to prescribe a combination medication and/or extended-release medication to decrease the number of pills taken.

Finally, educating the client can increase adherence. Clients who understand the purpose and importance of the prescription are more likely to be adherent.

Medication Safety Assessment, Reconciliation, and Management

As defined by the Joint Commission on Accreditation of Healthcare Organizations (JCAHO), medication reconciliation is "the process of comparing a patient's medication orders to all of the medications that the patient has been taking," including name, dosage, route, and frequency. Medications should also be checked for compatibility. It is important to review all prescribed medications, as well as over-the-counter medications and supplements, the patient is taking. As discussed in the previous section, the case manager should assess the client's understanding of why he is prescribed the medications and how to take them properly, as well as the client's compliance with taking the medications as ordered.

A case manager will rarely have a client who is not taking any medications. It is much more likely a client is taking multiple medications, for multiple conditions, prescribed by multiple providers. The goal of medication reconciliation is to decrease adverse drug events by reducing medication errors, such as omission, duplication, drug interactions, and dosing errors. Most errors occur during patient transitions in care, including changes in setting, level of care, or practitioner.

When Should Medication Reconciliation Occur?

- Any time the patient is moved within the hospital, such as from the ICU to the step down unit
- Upon transfer to another facility
- Upon discharge from any facility
- At each doctor office visit

Case managers should perform medication reconciliation upon opening the case, after each hospitalization, and after each visit to the doctor's office, at a minimum.

Transitions of Care/Transitional Care

Transitions of care can occur within a facility, such as when a patient is transferred from the ICU to the step-down unit; between facilities, such as from

a hospital to a skilled nursing facility; and within the community, from the primary care physician to the specialist.

A transitioning patient is at increased risk for an adverse outcome, due to medication errors, failure to follow up on testing or procedures, and/or not continuing prescribed treatments or therapies. Accountability—identifying who is responsible for what—is another concern. Failure to transition properly often occurs because of a communication breakdown. For this reason, the Centers for Medicare & Medicaid Services (CMS) recommends providers issue a summary of care for all transitions of care or referrals.

Public Health and Promoting Interoperability Programs (formerly Meaningful Use) is a CMS program that sets specific objectives that eligible professionals (EPs) and hospitals must achieve to qualify for Medicare and Medicaid Electronic Health Record (EHR) Incentive Programs. One of these objectives is the Electronic Exchanges of Summary of Care. This objective states that EPs who transition their patients to another setting of care or provider of care, or refer their patients to another provider of care, should provide a summary care record for each transition of care or referral.

For this objective, the term "transition of care" is defined as the movement of a patient from one setting of care (e.g., hospital, ambulatory primary care practice, specialty care practice, long-term care, home health care, or rehabilitation facility) to another. A summary of care record must include the following elements:

- Patient name
- Referring or transitioning provider's name and office contact information
- Procedures
- Encounter diagnosis
- Immunizations
- Laboratory test results
- Vital signs (height, weight, blood pressure, BMI)
- Smoking status
- Functional status, including activities of daily living, cognitive and disability status
- Demographic information (preferred language, sex, race, ethnicity, date of birth)
- Care plan field (at a minimum the following components must be included: problem-focus of the care plan, goal-target outcome, and any instructions that the provider has given to the patient)

- Care team, including the primary care provider of record and any additional known care team members beyond the referring or transitioning provider and the receiving provider
- Reason for the referral
- Current problem list (at minimum a list of current, active, and historical diagnoses, but the problem list is not limited to diagnoses)
- Current medication list
- Current medication allergy list
- Clinical importance

A transition of care summary, also known as a discharge summary in some circumstances, provides essential clinical information for the receiving care team and helps organize final clinical and administrative activities for the transferring care team. This summary helps ensure the coordination and continuity of healthcare as patients transfer between different locations or different levels of care within the same location. This document improves transitions and discharges, communication among providers, and cross-setting relationships, which can improve care quality and safety.

Transitions of care are such an important part of case management that The Commission for Case Manager Certification (CCMC) in their Case Management Body of Knowledge, lists both transitioning (transitional care) and communication post-transition as parts of the case management process. This is because the case manager is often involved during all points of transition and is in contact with the patient, family, and providers. This makes the case manager best suited to serve as coordinator of transitions of care.

**See Transitional Care and Post-transitional Communication in the Case Management Process and Tools section for more information.

Continuum of Care/Continuum of Health and Human/ Social Services

The continuum of care matches the ongoing needs of the individuals being served by the case management process with the appropriate level and type of health, medical, financial, legal, and psychosocial care for services within a setting or across multiple settings.

The role of the case manager varies depending on where the patient is in the healthcare continuum. In a non-acute setting, the focus may be on preventing illness or deterioration of illness. If the patient is in the acute setting, the case manager will coordinate care and/or services.

A case manager's role is to ensure continuity of care when a patient transitions through the continuum of care. The case manager is in a unique position to make certain that appropriate information is communicated to multiple providers to ensure a safe transition.

Interdisciplinary/Interprofessional Care Team

The Interdisciplinary Care Team and Interprofessional Care Team are both groups of healthcare professionals from various professional disciplines that work together to manage the physical, psychological, and spiritual needs of the patient. Whenever possible, the patient and the patient's family should be part of the team.

In an interdisciplinary team, each discipline creates its own assessment and treatment plan, evaluates the progress, and updates the plan independently. They may or may not report back to the interdisciplinary team.

The interprofessional team collaborates on a joint plan for the patient's assessment and treatment. Team members evaluate where there may be areas of role overlap and duplication, as well as gaps. The team collaborates to make optimal use of all collaborators. This team model works well with complex and chronic cases which require coordination among various disciplines with overlapping as well as unique contributions.

Members of the Interdisciplinary/Interprofessional Care Team may include:

- Physicians
- Nurses
- Case managers
- Social workers
- Physical therapists
- Occupational therapists
- Chaplains
- Dieticians
- Pharmacists

It is often the case manager's responsibility to assess the client's needs and the resources available. When the needs are identified, the case manager facilitates referrals to appropriate community-based providers and services.

Roles and Functions of Other Healthcare Providers in Various Care/Practice Settings

When referring a patient to a healthcare provider, the case manager should make sure the provider is professionally qualified to treat the patient.

Physician

The role of the physician is to improve the health and well-being of individuals by promoting, maintaining, or restoring health through diagnosis and treatment. The physician evaluates symptoms, performs tests, and prescribes medication or treatment for an illness or injury. He or she also counsels patients on how to prevent illness.

Nurse Practitioner

A nurse practitioner (NP) is an advanced practice nurse who helps with all aspects of patient care, including diagnosis, treatment, and consultations. In some states NPs can practice independently. Nurse practitioners can prescribe medications, including controlled substances, in all 50 states.

Certified Nurse Midwife

Certified nurse midwives care for childbearing women during preconception, prenatal, labor, delivery, and postpartum periods. They also provide family-planning counseling and gynecological care. They care for low-risk patients who desire a more natural and intervention-free childbirth experience.

Chiropractor

Chiropractors treat patients with health problems of the neuromusculoskeletal system, which includes nerves, bones, muscles, ligaments, and tendons. They use spinal adjustments, manipulation, and other techniques to manage the patient's health concerns, such as back and neck pain.

Speech-Language Pathologist

A speech-language pathologist or speech-language therapist assesses, diagnoses, treats, and helps prevent disorders of speech, language, cognitive-communication, voice, swallowing, fluency, and other related areas.

Certified Psychiatric Nurse Specialist

Certified psychiatric nurse specialists perform psychotherapy and manage medications for clients with behavioral health disorders.

Behavioral Health Counselor

A behavioral health counselor can perform counseling and psychotherapy services but cannot prescribe medication.

Clinical Psychologist

Clinical psychologists perform psychotherapy and psychological testing and counseling but cannot prescribe medication.

Psychiatrist

Psychiatrists treat people with more serious disorders requiring medication, such as major depression, attention deficit disorder, and bipolar disorder; they also perform psychotherapy and manage medication.

Hospice, Palliative, and End of Life Care

Hospice

Hospice provides comprehensive end of life care and support, including palliative care, to terminally ill patients and their families. The care provided by hospice extends beyond the patient's death by providing bereavement support to the family.

To qualify for hospice care, the patient's physician (if they have one) and hospice physician must document that the patient has a terminal illness that reduces life expectancy, usually to 6 months or less if the disease follows its normal course of progression.

Hospice care is a team approach, coordinated by a case manager. Depending on the medical plan, terminal illness, and related conditions, the plan of care and covered services can include any or all of these services:

- Physician services
- Nursing care
- Durable medical equipment
- Medical supplies (like bandages and catheters)
- Prescription drugs related to the hospice diagnosis
- Hospice aide and homemaker services
- Physical and occupational therapy
- Speech-language pathology services
- Social worker services
- Dietary counseling
- Grief and loss counseling for the patient and family
- Short-term inpatient care (for pain and symptom management)
- Short-term respite care

Not covered under the hospice benefit is room and board and treatment to cure the disease.

Hospice care can be provided in a freestanding hospice facility or the patient's home. "Home" is wherever the patient lives and does not need to be a traditional home; it can be an assisted living facility, nursing home, homeless shelter, or any other place the patient calls home.

The hospice case manager's goals are unique to each patient but frequently include:

- Control of pain and other symptoms, giving the patient a better quality of life
- Provide the patient and family information they need to make informed decisions regarding treatment and the plan of care to ensure the patient has a dignified death
- Coordination and facilitation of care

A Do Not Resuscitate (DNR) is not necessary before enrolling in hospice, but patients and families are educated on this topic, with the goal of having the DNR in place before a patient's death.

Tools used to assess for hospice appropriateness:

Karnofsky Performance Scale – Measures performance status on a scale of 0-100%, with 0 being deceased and 100 being normal with no complications. A score of less than 70% (cares for self but is unable to carry on normal activities or work) can be one of the criteria for hospice.

Eastern Cooperative Oncology Group (ECOG) Performance Status Scale – A 0-4 scale with 0 being fully active and 4 completely disabled.

Palliative Performance Scale (PPS) – Uses five observer-rated domains (ambulation, activity level/evidence of disease, self-care, intake, and level of consciousness) correlated to the Karnofsky Performance Scale (0-100). It is a reliable tool that aids in determining appropriateness for hospice, especially for cancer patients.

Hospice care is a covered benefit for Medicare, Medicaid in most states, most private insurance companies, and many HMOs. The case manager should check the individual's hospice benefit for private insurance and HMOs, as benefits will vary.

**See more on the Medicare and Medicaid Hospice Benefits under Public Benefits Programs.

Palliative Care

Many people use the terms palliative care and hospice interchangeably, but there are important distinctions to make. Palliative care can be employed with a patient at any stage of a severe illness. It can be used concurrently with curative treatment. Palliative care is not dependent on prognosis. Alternatively, hospice care provides comprehensive care, including palliative care, for terminally ill patients with a life expectancy of six months or less, who are no longer receiving curative treatment.

Palliative care is specialized medical care for patients suffering from serious and chronic illnesses, such as cancer, CHF, COPD, kidney failure, and ALS, just to name a few. The goal of palliative care is for the patient and his family to maintain the best quality of life possible, by managing symptoms such as pain, fatigue, dyspnea, constipation, nausea, anorexia, and depression. Palliative care can be given alongside other medical treatments, such as chemotherapy and radiation, and can improve the ability to tolerate those treatments.

To achieve the goal of symptom management, some medication dosages and routes of administration may be different from the standard. It is also not uncommon for medications to be used off label. For example, anticonvulsants may be used to treat pain, or morphine to ease dyspnea.

Palliative care is a team approach, with the core team including the doctor, nurse, and social worker. Other members may be brought onto the team as needed, including a chaplain, pharmacist, dietitian, massage therapist, or music therapist, among others. The palliative care team works together with the patient's other doctors and providers to anticipate, prevent, and treat suffering. The majority of palliative care today is provided by hospice, although there are palliative care specialists and practices.

End of Life Care

About 25% of all Medicare spending is used to provide care in the beneficiary's last year of life. Case managers can help clients and families make informed decisions regarding end of life care that can prevent or relieve suffering and make an impact on the costs that are associated with end of life care. The case manager should understand the client's wishes regarding end of life care. Once these wishes are understood, the case manager can provide education as to the options available and how to ensure the client's wishes are acted on. This could be in the form of a palliative care consult, hospice, and/or advance directives such as a durable power of attorney, living will, and/or do not resuscitate.

Patient Self-Determination Act

The Patient Self-Determination Act (PSDA) amends titles XVIII (Medicare) and XIX (Medicaid) of the Social Security Act. It requires all hospitals, skilled nursing facilities, home health agencies, hospice programs, and health maintenance organizations that receive Medicare and Medicaid reimbursement to recognize the living will and durable power of attorney for healthcare. Under the PSDA they must:

- Ask patients if they have an advance directive
- Inform the patient of their rights under state law to make decisions concerning their medical care
- Not discriminate against persons who have executed an advance directive
- Ensure legally valid advance directives are implemented to the extent permitted by state law
- Provide education programs for staff, patients, and the community on ethical issues concerning patient self-determination and advance directives

Advance Directives

- Advance directives come in two forms: those that dictate what kind of medical treatment to be given or withheld such as a living will or do not resuscitate; and those that appoint an agent or proxy to make healthcare decisions. Both forms only go into effect if the person is unable to make the decision for themself. All states have their own advance directive forms and requirements. Next, is a description of the different types of advance directives available. It is important to note that the names may vary slightly between states and organizations.

Living Will

A living will states which specific medical treatments the designated person would like to receive or have withheld. These treatments can include, but are not limited to:

- Mechanical ventilation
- Dialysis
- Tube feedings
- IV fluids
- Antibiotics
- CPR

Healthcare Power of Attorney

This type of advance directive stipulates who is to make healthcare decisions for the person if they are unable to make decisions for themselves.

Do Not Resuscitate/Do Not Attempt Resuscitation/Allow Natural Death

A do not resuscitate (DNR), do not attempt resuscitation (DNAR), or allow natural death (AND) is another type of advance directive that is a request not to have CPR attempted.

BONUS

Although not required, I highly recommend you access the free 7-day Email Mini Course that I've created for you, which you can access at

CCMcertificationMadeEasy.com

In this free course, you'll get access to a step-by-step process including video instructions that will allow you to create a study plan that meets your individual needs.

References

Case Management Society of America. (2016). *Standards of practice for case management.* http://solutions.cmsa.org/acton/media/10442/standards-of-practice-for-case-management

Case Management Society of America & National Association of Social Workers. (2008). *Case management caseload concept paper.* http://api.cmsa.org:8080/Individual/MemberResources/CaseloadConceptPaperMatrix/tabid/363/Default.aspx

Centers for Medicare & Medicaid Services. (n.d.). https://www.cms.gov/

Centers for Medicare & Medicaid Services. (2020, March). *Medicare hospice benefits.* https://ccmcertification.org/get-certified/exam-study-materials/ccmc-glossary

Commission for Case Management Certification. (n.d.). *Case management body of knowledge.* https://cmbodyofknowledge.com/

Commission for Case Management Certification. (2017). *Glossary of terms.* https://ccmcertification.org/get-certified/exam-study-materials/ccmc-glossary

Commission for Case Management Certification. (n.d.). *Case management philosophy and guiding principles.* Case Management Body of Knowledge. https://cmbodyofknowledge.com/content/case-management-philosophy-and-guiding-principles

Dorland Health. (2013). *The caseload guidebook for successful outcomes.* https://www.dorlandhealth.com

Kessler, R.C. (1990-1992 Restricted Version). *National comorbidity survey: Baseline (NCS-1).* Inter-University Consortium for Political and Social Research, 2009.

Kleinsinger, F. (2018, Jul 5). The unmet challenge of medication nonadherence. *The Permanente Journal,* 22:18-033. https://doi.org/10.7812/TPP/18-033

The Joint Commission. (n.d.). https://www.jointcommission.org/

Chapter Three:
Care Delivery and
Reimbursement Methods
Part 2

Care Delivery and Reimbursement Methods comprises 28% of the exam with between 40 and 44 questions on this topic. It is the largest area of the exam. This has been divided into two parts for easier reading.

****

A case manager must have a broad knowledge of care delivery and reimbursement methods to perform her job effectively. She must understand the clinical and financial resources available to her client, as well as the eligibility criteria for receiving those resources. This will enable her to ensure the client receives the most appropriate care in a cost-effective manner.

Financial Resources

The diagnosis of a serious or terminal illness can be financially devastating for an individual and his family. Often the patient can no longer work and the medical bills mount, quickly depleting a person's entire life savings. The following are financial resources that may be available.

Waiver Programs

Medicaid Waiver programs provide long-term care services at home and in the community to people who would otherwise be in an institution, nursing home, or hospital. Prior to the waivers, the federal Medicaid program only paid for long-term care services provided in an institution.

Waiver programs can provide a combination of standard medical services and non-medical services. Standard services include but are not limited to case management, homemaker, home health aide, personal care, adult day health services, habilitation (both day and residential), assisted living, and respite care. States can also propose other services that may assist in diverting and/or transitioning individuals from institutional settings into their homes and communities.

The Katie Beckett Waiver enables severely disabled children and adults to be cared for at home and to be eligible for Medicaid based on the affected individual's income and assets alone. Before the Katie Beckett Waiver, the income of legally liable relatives was counted when the individual was cared for at home.

Special Needs Trusts

A trust is a relationship between three parties: a donor who contributes the funds for the trust, a trustee who manages and administers the funds according to the donor's wishes, and a beneficiary who receives the funds. A special needs trust (SNT) is designed for beneficiaries who are disabled, either physically or mentally. SNTs can be tailored to meet the unique circumstances of each family.

Types of SNTs include General Support and Supplemental Care. The General Support SNT is designed to be the primary or sole source of benefits for the beneficiary. This type of trust is considered an available resource of the beneficiary and can make him ineligible for needs-based benefits. The Supplemental Care SNT is designed as a secondary source of benefits for the beneficiary after governmental benefits have been exhausted. A properly prepared Supplemental Care SNT will allow the beneficiary to be eligible for need-based government benefits, such as Medicaid and Supplemental Security Income, while still receiving funds from the trust.

Accelerated Death Benefit

Some life insurance policies have an accelerated death benefit (ADB) rider, allowing an insured person with a terminal illness to use some of the policy's benefit prior to dying. The ADB is deducted from the amount the beneficiaries receive at death. There are restrictions on how the money can be used; generally, it can be used for long-term care and medical expenses.

Viatical Settlements

A life insurance policy is personal property, meaning it can be sold. A viatical settlement sells the life insurance policy of a person with a terminal or life-threatening illness and a life expectancy of less than five years to a third party for cash. There are no restrictions on how this money can be used. The purchasing party then becomes the beneficiary and takes responsibility for paying the premium.

The insured is normally paid between 50-80% of the face value of the policy. This amount is dependent on a number of factors, such as life expectancy, current interest rates, and the cost of paying the premium.

Due to HIPAA protections, the money received from a viatical settlement is usually free from federal income tax. However, earnings may impact eligibility for some means-based programs such as Medicaid.

Reverse Mortgages

A reverse mortgage may be an option for a patient who is a homeowner and age 62 or older. Under a reverse mortgage, the patient borrows against his home's value without having to leave the home or make payments. The funds can be distributed by:

- Lump sum
- Fixed monthly installments
- Line of credit

The payment structure of the proceeds may impact Medicaid eligibility. The line of credit is the most popular choice and often is not considered an asset when determining Medicaid eligibility.

The amount of money received through a reverse mortgage is determined by the home's value, the age of the borrower, and current interest rates. There are no restrictions on how the money can be used. The loan does not have to be repaid until the last borrower dies, sells the house, or moves out.

A reverse mortgage is not for everyone. Both spouses must be 62 or older to be listed on the reverse mortgage deed. If only one spouse is listed, and he or she dies first, the surviving spouse must repay the loan in full or be evicted.

Employer-Based Health and Wellness Programs

An employer-based health and wellness program is an extra benefit provided to employees, and sometimes their dependents, to improve their health and well being. This can be in the form of preventive care as well as behavioral change interventions, medical screenings, incentives, fitness programs, social support, or competitions.

The goals of these programs can include improving employees' motivation and morale, improving employees' quality of life, and preventing and managing chronic diseases to lower their economic and health burden. Decreasing modifiable health risk factors, and thereby decreasing the incidence of chronic disease and disability, should result in healthier employees, lower health care and health insurance costs, reduced absenteeism, and increased productivity.

Some examples of these programs include:

- Stress reduction programs
- Weight loss programs
- Wellness challenges (walking challenge, water challenge)
- Smoking cessation programs
- Health risk assessments
- Health screenings
- Exercise program and activities
- Onsite fitness center
- Nutrition education
- Vaccination clinic
- Employee assistance program (EAP)

Employee assistance programs (EAPs) generally offer free and confidential assessments, short-term counseling, referrals, and follow-up services for employees and possibly their dependents. Support can be provided for numerous issues or areas of concern including stress, substance abuse, depression, anxiety, legal counseling, financial concerns, aging parents, healthcare concerns, and family and personal relationship issues. EAPs are a great resource for case managers to refer clients for additional support.

Case managers who work in employer-based health and wellness programs will need to demonstrate the effectiveness of the program, as well as the value it brings to the organization. A baseline will need to be established as well as the metrics used to evaluate the effectiveness and value.

Insurance Principles (e.g., health, disability, workers' compensation, long-term care)

Health Insurance

CCMC defines health insurance as, "Protection which provides payment of benefits for coverage for covered sickness or injury. Included under this heading are various types of insurance such as accident insurance, disability income insurance, medical expense insurance, and accidental death and dismemberment insurance" (CCMC Glossary of Terms, 2017).

Medical expense insurance provides payment of benefits for covered sickness or injury as well as some preventive care. Traditional medical insurance only covers medical expenses that are considered "medically necessary." What is deemed medically necessary varies by health plan.

In general, medically necessary services are those that are reasonable, necessary, appropriate, and based on evidence-based standards of care. Cosmetic procedures are usually not considered medically necessary. Home modifications, caregivers, healthy meals, transportation to doctor appointments and treatments, and long term care are not normally covered by medical insurance.

Coordination of Benefits (COB)

To prevent double payment for medical services when a subscriber has coverage from two or more sources, the National Association of Insurance Commissioners created COB guidelines. Following these guidelines is not mandatory, but most states and commercial insurances choose to use these COB provisions to determine which insurer is primary and which is secondary.

The primary plan is initially responsible for payment of benefits for covered services as if there were no other plan. After the primary plan has paid, the balance is passed to the secondary company, which pays according to its contract.

The following determines which plan is primary:

- Medicaid always pays last.
- If an insurance plan does not have a COB provision, it must pay primary.
- If none of the below applies, the coverage that has been in force the longest is primary.

Employees

- The insurance plan covering the client as an employee is the primary payer over a plan covering the individual as a dependent.
- The insurance plan that covers an active employee is primary over the plan that covers a retiree or laid-off employee.
- The insurance plan that covers an active employee is primary over a COBRA plan.

Dependents of married parents

- If the parents are married, the birthday rule states that the parent whose birthday comes first in the year is primary for the children.

Dependents of non-married parents

- If the parents are not married and both plans cover the client as a dependent, primary coverage is determined by the court.
- If no court determination has been made, the parent with custody is primary, followed by the spouse of the parent with custody, and finally the parent without custody.

Medicare

- Age 65 or older and **retired**, Medicare is primary.
- Age 65 or older and covered due to the patient or his spouse working for an employer with **20 or more employees**, the employer plan is primary.
- Age 65 or older and covered due to the patient or spouse working for an employer with **fewer than 20 employees**, Medicare is primary.

- Under age 65 and disabled, and covered on the patient or family member's current employer plan with **100 or more employees**, the employer plan is primary.

- Under age 65 and disabled, and covered on the patient or family member's current employer plan with **fewer than 100 employees**, Medicare is primary.

- Medicare based on ESRD and also on a group health plan, the group plan is primary for the first 30 months after eligibility to enroll in Medicare. Medicare is primary after the first 30 months.

Long-Term Care Insurance

Traditional insurance and Medicare do not pay for long-term care (LTC). A long-term care policy may offset some or all of the cost of long-term care. These policies vary widely, but usually have a limit on the dollar amount or number of years one can receive the benefit.

Some policies cover care in the patient's home, while others only cover care in a facility. Depending on the LTC company, the patient may be able to hire independent providers or family members to care for them. Other companies require the patient to use a certified agency or licensed providers. Some of the services that may be covered include adult day care, home care, home modifications, assisted living, and nursing home.

Workers' Compensation

Workers' compensation laws protect employees who are injured or disabled on the job. They are designed to provide fixed monetary awards, eliminating the need for litigation. Workers covered by workers' compensation cannot sue their employer for work-related injuries. Benefits include both medical costs and lost wages, and are awarded to the worker regardless of who was at fault for the accident.

The employer is 100% responsible for paying for workers' compensation insurance. The employer is also responsible for filing the First Report of Injury with the insurance carrier and the state workers' compensation agency, if required. In addition to covering injured and disabled workers, workers' compensation also provides benefits for dependents of workers killed by work-related accidents or illnesses.

Workers' compensation regulations vary from state to state, and state mandates take precedence over the financial status or will of the employer. Federal statutes are limited to federal employees or those workers employed in some significant aspect of interstate commerce.

Federal Workers' Compensation Programs

Federal Employment Compensation Act – Provides workers' compensation for non-military federal employees.

Federal Employment Liability Act (FELA) – Ensures that railroads engaged in interstate commerce are liable for injuries to their employees if they have been negligent.

Merchant Marine Act (aka the Jones Act) – Provides seamen with the same protection from employer negligence as FELA provides for railroad workers.

Longshore and Harbor Workers' Compensation Act (LHWCA) – Provides workers' compensation to specified employees of private maritime employers.

Black Lung Benefits Act – Provides compensation for miners suffering from "black lung." The Act requires liable mine operators to pay disability payments. It also establishes a fund that provides disability payments to miners when the mine operator is unknown or unable to pay.

Workers' compensation pays for:

- Medical care that is considered "reasonable and customary" for work-related injuries, beginning immediately after the injury occurs
- Temporary disability benefits
- Permanent partial and permanent total disability benefits to workers who have lasting consequences of disabilities caused on the job
- Rehabilitation and training benefits for those unable to return to pre-injury career
- Benefits to survivors of workers who die of work-related causes

Claims Management Strategies

Workers' compensation always pays primary to short-term disability (STD), long-term disability (LTD), and Social Security Disability Insurance (SSDI).

When considering the award amount for loss of income or earning capacity due to an occupational injury, disease, or death, the following classifications of disability are used:

- Temporary Total Disability (TTD) – The worker is totally incapacitated for work beyond the day on which the accident occurred but is subsequently able to return to work. The majority of workers' compensation injuries fall under this classification.
- Permanent Total Disability (PTD) – The injury permanently and totally incapacitates the injured worker from carrying out gainful employment.
- Temporary Partial Disability (TPD) – The worker is partially incapacitated for the length of the disability. Although unable to perform normal work duties, he may engage in modified work.
- Permanent Partial Disability (PPD) – The worker has a partial loss of function that does not prevent work and is permanent.

Disability Income Insurance

CCMC defines disability income insurance as a form of health insurance that provides periodic payment to replace income when an insured person is unable to work as a result of illness, injury, or disease.

Workers' compensation, short-term disability insurance (STD), long-term disability insurance (LTD), and Social Security Disability Insurance (SSDI) benefits all provide financial compensation for workers who are unable to work. There are differences between the programs, however. Workers' compensation only covers work-related injuries, while STD and LTD cover loss of work due to illness, injury, or accident that is not work-related.

Workers' compensation provides replacement of lost wages and a medical benefit for the work-related injury. STD and LTD only cover a portion of the wages, typically 50-70%, and begin after a waiting period.

Workers' compensation premiums are mandated to be paid by the employer. The employer can also provide LTD and STD as part of a benefits package, or an individual can purchase LTD and/or STD policies from an agent. LTD purchased from an agent is not taxed, whereas LTD as part of a benefits package is taxed. SSDI is paid for by a tax on the employer and the employee.

**SSDI is covered in greater detail in the section Public Benefits Programs.

Disability Comparison

	WC	STD	LTD	SSDI
Wage Replacement	Yes	Yes, a portion	Yes, a portion	Yes, amount depends on work record
Medical Benefit	Yes	No	No	Medicare is available after 24 months of receiving SSDI
Work Related	Yes	Covers non-work related injury, accident, or illness	Covers non-work related injury, accident, or illness	Covers non-work related injury, accident, or illness
Paid By	Employer	Employer, employee, or both	Employer, employee, or both	Funded by Social Security taxes paid by workers, employers, and the self-employed
Waiting Period	No	Yes, usually 7-30 days (and ends 90-180 days after day of disability)	Yes, LTD usually begins after STD ends	5-month waiting period

Private Benefit Programs

Employer-sponsored Health Coverage

Employer-sponsored health insurance is coverage offered by an employer to its employees. Employers can choose to purchase a fully-insured plan and pay a fixed premium to an insurance carrier or choose to self-insure the health plan.

With a fully-insured plan, the premium cost is set for the year. The insurance carrier collects the premium and pays the claims as outlined in the policy.

Some employers choose to self-fund their health plans in an attempt to reduce costs. Self-funded, or self-insured, employers do not pay a fixed premium to an insurance carrier. Instead, they pay for each claim as it is incurred, out of pocket. To do this, they must meet the state's legal and financial requirements.

Self-insured employers may purchase reinsurance, excess risk, or stop-loss insurance to offset very large claims. Employers that self-insure often contract with third-party administrators (TPAs) or administrative services only (ASOs) to handle the administrative aspects of insurance, such as utilization review and processing claims. Self-funded plans are regulated federally by ERISA (Employee Retirement Income Security Act of 1974) and are exempt from most laws regulating fully-insured plans on the state level.

Individual-purchased Insurance

Individual health insurance is purchased on an individual or family basis, as opposed to being provided by the employer. Individual health insurance policies are regulated by the state in which they are purchased. The Patient Protection and Affordable Care Act (ACA) has made significant changes to how individual policies are rated and the benefits that these policies provide. All policies must cover the same set of Essential Health Benefits. The ACA also subsidizes policies purchased through the exchanges for certain qualified individuals.

Indemnity

CCMC defines indemnity benefits as "benefits in the form of payments rather than services." In most cases, this means the healthcare provider bills the patient, and the insurance company reimburses the patient later. Indemnity benefits are also known as fee-for-service. The patient is free to choose his provider without restriction, but indemnity policies are more expensive than managed care policies.

Pharmacy Benefit Management

Pharmacy benefit management services use a number of strategies to control the cost of prescription medications. One such strategy is contracting with a network of retail pharmacies to provide discounted rates for members. They may also use mail-order pharmacies, through which medications are mailed to the patient's home at a savings over retail prices. Pharmacy benefit management services use their large purchasing power to negotiate discounts from drug manufacturers. They also develop and maintain a formulary—a list of drugs approved for reimbursement—to encourage the use of lower cost drugs. Pharmacy benefit management services often use payment tiers, with generic drugs being the cheapest, followed by formulary medications, and then non-formulary medications. Other strategies include implementing step therapy, quantity restrictions on certain classes of drugs, and prior-authorization.

Home Care Benefits

Most benefit plans include home care. The extent of the benefit varies, so the case manager should be aware of the limitations on this benefit. There may be limits on the number of visits per year, the number of hours per visit, and/or the types of services that may be provided.

COBRA

In 1986, Congress passed the Consolidated Omnibus Budget Reconciliation Act (COBRA). Under this law, employees and their families (spouse, former spouse, and dependent children) who might otherwise lose their health insurance due to certain events can choose to keep their insurance. The events include:

- A covered employee's death,
- A covered employee's job loss or reduction in hours for any reasons other than gross misconduct,
- A covered employee becomes entitled to Medicare,

- A covered employee's divorce or legal separation, and
- A child's loss of dependent status (and therefore coverage) under the plan.

Employers (private sector or state/local government) with 20 or more employees offer COBRA.

If a person elects COBRA coverage, he continues to receive group health benefits from the plan for a limited period of time. The duration of coverage under COBRA is usually 18 months. But there are two circumstances which can extend coverage. The first is when one of the qualified beneficiaries is disabled; the second is when a second qualifying event occurs.

Extension Due to Disability

If one of the qualified beneficiaries in a family is disabled and meets certain requirements, all of the qualified beneficiaries in that family are entitled to an 11-month extension of the maximum period of continuation coverage (for a total maximum period of 29 months of continuation coverage). The plan can charge qualified beneficiaries an increased premium, up to 150 percent of the cost of coverage, during the 11-month disability extension.

The requirements are:

1. the Social Security Administration (SSA) determines that the qualified beneficiary is disabled before the 60th day of continuation coverage; and

2. the disability continues for the duration of the initial 18-month period of continuation coverage.

Extension Due to Second Qualifying Event

An 18-month extension may be available to qualified beneficiaries receiving an 18-month maximum period of continuation coverage (giving a total maximum period of 36 months of continuation coverage) if the qualified beneficiaries experience a second qualifying event, for example, death of the covered employee, divorce or legal separation of the covered employee and spouse, Medicare entitlement (in certain circumstances), or loss of dependent child status under the plan.

Summary of Qualifying Events, Qualified Beneficiaries, and Maximum Periods of Continuation Coverage

The following chart shows the maximum period for which continuation coverage must be offered for the specific qualifying events and the qualified beneficiaries who are entitled to elect continuation coverage when the specific event occurs. **Note that an event is a qualifying event only if it causes the qualified beneficiary to lose coverage under the plan.**

QUALIFYING EVENT	QUALIFIED BENEFICIARIES	MAXIMUM PERIOD OF CONTINUATION COVERAGE
Termination (for reasons other than gross misconduct) or reduction in hours of employment	Employee Spouse Dependent Child	18 months [*]
Employee enrollment in Medicare	Spouse Dependent Child	36 months [*]
Divorce or legal separation	Spouse Dependent Child	36 months
Death of employee	Spouse Dependent Child	36 months
Loss of "dependent child" status under the plan	Dependent Child	36 months

*See exceptions on extensions previously mentioned in text.

Note: Reprinted from, "An employer's guide to group health continuation coverage under COBRA," by Employee Benefits Security Administration, 2018, p.11. Retrieved from https://www.dol.gov/sites/dolgov/files/EBSA/about-ebsa/our-activities/resource-center/publications/an-employers-guide-to-group-health-continuation-coverage-under-cobra.pdf

The eligible person must elect COBRA within 60 days of the termination of plan coverage. After the initial election, the first premium payment must be made within 45 days. After this, payments are due on the first of each month, subject to a 30-day grace period. If payments are not made as stated, coverage may be terminated.

Group health plans can require qualified beneficiaries to pay for COBRA continuation coverage, although plans can choose to provide continuation coverage at reduced or no cost. In calculating premiums for continuation coverage, a plan can include the costs paid by both the employee and the employer, plus an additional two percent for administrative costs. As stated previously, for qualified beneficiaries receiving the 11-month disability extension of continuation coverage, the premium for those additional months may be increased to 150 percent of the plan's total cost of coverage. This makes COBRA financially out of reach for many of the people who qualify for it (Employer's Guide to Group Health Continuation Coverage Under COBRA, 2018).

Public Benefit Programs

Public benefits programs include Social Security Disability Insurance (SSDI), Supplemental Security Income (SSI), Medicare, and Medicaid. Individuals who are entitled to both Medicare and Medicaid are called dual eligibles. In the case of dual eligibles, Medicaid always pays last.

MEDICARE

Medicare is health insurance provided by the U.S. Government for people who are 65 or older, certain younger people with disabilities, and people with End Stage Renal Disease (ESRD). It was created in 1966 under Title XVIII of the Social Security Act and is administered by the Centers for Medicare & Medicaid Services (CMS). Medicare covers some but not all medical costs and pays under the Prospective Payment System (PPS) for most care settings.

Medicare eligibility is not based on income. However, the premiums for Part B and Part D will be higher for certain income groups. This is known as income-related monthly adjustment amount, or IRMAA, and is a surcharge that high-income people may pay in addition to their Medicare Part B and Part D premiums.

Eligibility for Medicare benefits:

- 65 or older, or
- Have a specific long-term disability (and have been receiving Social Security Disability benefits for at least 24 months), or
- Have Lou Gehrig's disease (the waiting period is also waived), or
- Diagnosed with permanent kidney failure (ESRD), requiring dialysis or transplant

Medicare has 4 parts:

- Part A (Hospital Insurance)
- Part B (Medical Insurance)
- Part C (Medicare Advantage Plan)
- Part D (Prescription Drugs)

Medicare Part A

Medicare Part A pays for:

- Inpatient hospital stays, including acute care hospitals, critical access hospitals, inpatient rehabilitation facilities, and long-term care hospitals
- Skilled nursing facility stays
- Home health care
- Hospice care

It is important to note that not all overnight hospital stays are inpatient stays. To qualify as an inpatient, the patient must pass CMS's Two-Midnight rule. This rule is a Medicare payment policy regarding the benchmark criteria to use when determining whether inpatient admission is reasonable and necessary for purposes of payment under Medicare Part A.

In general, the Two-Midnight rule states that inpatient admissions are generally payable under Part A if the admitting practitioner expects the patient to require a hospital stay that crosses two midnights and the medical record supports that reasonable expectation.

A patient that does not meet the criteria for inpatient admission will be placed in observation status which is paid under Medicare Part B. This has numerous implications including:

- A beneficiary usually pays a copayment for each outpatient hospital service he receives, as well as 20% of the Medicare-approved amount for most doctor services after the Part B deductible is met.
- Medicare Part A will only cover SNF care if the beneficiary had a 3-day minimum, medically necessary inpatient hospital stay for a related illness or injury.
- Prescription and over-the-counter drugs a beneficiary receives in a hospital outpatient setting aren't covered by Part B. If the beneficiary has a Medicare prescription drug plan (Part D), the plan may help pay for these drugs, but the beneficiary will need to pay out-of-pocket for these drugs and submit a claim to the drug plan for a refund.

A "Medicare Outpatient Observation Notice" (MOON) is a document that must be given to a Medicare patient who is receiving observation or outpatient services for more than 24 hours to let them know they are an outpatient (and not an inpatient) in a hospital or critical access hospital.

Some individuals must pay a premium for Medicare Part A, but most people are covered for free. To be eligible for premium-free Part A, an individual must be entitled to receive Medicare based on their own earnings or those of a spouse, parent, or child. The worker must have a specified number of quarters of coverage (QCs), usually 40 quarters or 10 years. The exact number of QCs required depends on whether the person is filing for Part A coverage on the basis of age, disability, or ESRD. Individuals can check their status by contacting the Social Security Administration prior to retirement. QCs are earned through payment of payroll taxes under the Federal Insurance Contributions Act (FICA) during the person's working years.

Those who are not eligible for premium-free part A may be able to buy Part A. To be eligible to purchase Part A, an individual must be age 65 or older and be enrolled in Medicare Part B. They will be required to pay a premium for both Parts A and B.

Inpatient Hospital Coverage Under Medicare Part A

Medicare covers up to 90 days of medically necessary inpatient hospital care per benefit period. The beneficiary is responsible for the initial deductible and a copayment based on when in the benefit period they are hospitalized.

Benefit Periods
- A benefit period begins when the beneficiary is first admitted to the hospital. It ends when the patient has been out of the hospital or skilled nursing facility for at least 60 consecutive days.
- There is no limit to the number of benefit periods covered during a beneficiary's lifetime.
- Inpatient hospital care is normally limited to 90 days during a benefit period.
- Deductible is required for days 1-60 of each benefit period.
- Copayment is required for days 61-90.
- If the 90 days are exhausted, the beneficiary can elect to use days from a non-renewable "lifetime reserve" of up to 60 additional days of inpatient hospital care. (Copayment is also required for these days.)
- The patient is responsible for all costs for each day after all lifetime reserve days are used.

Skilled Nursing Facility (SNF) Coverage Under Medicare Part A

Medicare Part A covers semi-private rooms, meals, skilled nursing and rehabilitative services, and other medically necessary services and supplies furnished in a skilled nursing facility only if it is within 30 days of an inpatient hospital stay of 3 days or more for a related illness or injury and is medically necessary. Coverage of skilled nursing care or skilled therapy care is only covered if it is necessary to improve or maintain the patient's current condition.

To qualify for skilled nursing facility care coverage, the patient must need daily skilled care (like intravenous fluids/medications or physical therapy), which can only be provided as an inpatient of a skilled nursing facility. Medicare doesn't cover long-term care or custodial care.

There is no copayment for the first 20 days of each benefit period. Days 21-100 have a daily copayment. There is a limit of 100 days per benefit period, after that the patient is 100% responsible for payment.

Home Health Care Under Medicare Part A

Medicare covers medically necessary:

- Part-time or intermittent skilled nursing care
- Physical therapy
- Speech-language pathology services
- Occupational therapy services
- Medical social services
- Part-time or intermittent home health aide services, if intermittent or part time skilled nursing and/or other therapy or rehabilitation is provided

Full-time nursing is not covered. Medicare Part A covers the first 100 visits following a 3-day hospitalization or SNF stay, and there is no copayment or deductible. To qualify for home care the patient must be "homebound," which means:

- They have trouble leaving home without help (like using a cane, wheelchair, walker, or crutches; special transportation; or help from another person) because of an illness or injury.

- Leaving home isn't recommended because of their condition.

- They are normally unable to leave home because it's a major effort.

Medicare Hospice Benefit

Eligibility for the Medicare Hospice Benefit:

- The patient has Medicare Part A

- The hospice program is Medicare approved

- The patient will no longer receive curative care for the terminal illness or related conditions

- The client's regular physician (if they have one) and hospice physician certify that the patient has a life expectancy of six months or less if the illness runs its normal course

What Medicare Hospice Benefit Covers

Medicare covers a one-time-only hospice consultation with a hospice medical director or hospice doctor to discuss care options. This is covered even if the client decides not to proceed with hospice care.

Once the hospice benefit starts, Original Medicare will cover everything related to the terminal illness as long as it is coordinated by the hospice provider including:

- Physician services

- Nursing care

- Durable medical equipment

- Medical supplies (like bandages and catheters)

- Prescription drugs related to the hospice diagnosis

- Hospice aide and homemaker services
- Physical and occupational therapy
- Speech-language pathology services
- Social worker services
- Dietary counseling
- Grief and loss counseling for the patient and family
- Short-term inpatient care (for pain and symptom management)
- Short-term (up to 5 days) of respite care provided at a Medicare-approved facility (like a hospice inpatient facility, hospital, or nursing home)
- Any other Medicare-covered services needed to manage the terminal illness and related conditions, as recommended by the hospice team

What Medicare Hospice Benefit Doesn't Cover

- Treatment intended to cure the terminal illness and/or related conditions
- Prescription drugs not related to the terminal illness or related conditions
- Care from any provider that wasn't set up by the hospice medical team
- Room and board, other than short-term inpatient or respite care services that are approved and arranged by the hospice team
- Hospital outpatient, emergency department, or inpatient care unless it is either arranged by the hospice team or is unrelated to the terminal illness
- Ambulance transportation, unless it's either arranged by the hospice team or is unrelated to the terminal illness and related conditions

Cost of Medicare Hospice Care

Medicare patients who elect the hospice benefit have minimal to no out-of-pocket expenses for most hospice services. There is no deductible for hospice care. The only cost-sharing responsibilities come from a 5% coinsurance for inpatient respite care, if used, and a copayment of up to $5 per outpatient prescription drug. They are required to continue paying their monthly Medicare Part A (hospital) and Part B (Medical) insurance premiums.

Care for a Condition Other Than the Terminal Illness

After the hospice benefit starts, the patient can still get covered services for conditions not related to the terminal illness. Original Medicare will pay for covered services for any health problems that aren't part of the terminal illness and related conditions. However, the patient will be responsible for the deductible and coinsurance amounts for all Medicare-covered services obtained to treat health problems that aren't part of the terminal illness and related conditions. If the patient was on a Medicare Advantage Plan before starting hospice care, and decided to stay in that plan, they can get covered services for any health problems that aren't part of their terminal illness and related conditions. They can choose to get these from either their Medicare Advantage Plan or Original Medicare.

Benefit Periods

Hospice care is given in benefit periods. The first and second benefit periods are 90 days each. These periods are followed by unlimited 60-day benefit periods. At the start of each benefit period, a physician must certify that the patient is terminally ill. The patient may change hospice providers once during a benefit period.

Medicare Part B

Medicare Part B is voluntary insurance; there is a monthly premium for coverage. It pays for:

- Physician and surgeon services
- Outpatient services
- Durable medical equipment*
- Mental health services
- Ambulance
- Emergency room care

- Preventive services
- Home health care*

*Medicare Part B covers home health care not associated with a hospital or SNF stay. It also covers after the 100 days covered under Part A. There is no copayment or deductible for home health. Durable medical equipment has 80/20 cost-sharing, known as a copayment, where Medicare will cover 80% of the cost and the beneficiary is responsible for the remaining 20%.

Medicare Part B has a deductible that may apply to some services. After the deductible is met, Medicare will pay 80% of the Medicare-approved amount, and the patient is responsible for the 20% coinsurance. There is no out-of-pocket limit.

Medicare Part C (Medicare Advantage Plan)

Medicare Advantage Plans are a managed care option to obtain coverage for Parts A and B and sometimes D, through a private health plan such as an HMO, PPO, Special Needs Plan (SNP), HMO Point of Service (HMOPOS) plan, or Medicare Medical Savings Account plan.

Most Medicare Advantage Plans offer coverage for things that are not covered by Original Medicare, like vision, hearing, dental, and wellness programs (like gym memberships). Plans can also cover services like transportation to doctor visits, over-the-counter drugs, adult day care services, and other health-related services that promote health and wellness. In addition, plans can tailor their benefit packages to offer new benefits to certain chronically ill enrollees. These packages will provide benefits customized to treat those conditions.

- Plans contract with the government to administer Medicare benefits to members.
- Plans are required to provide services covered in Medicare Parts A and B except hospice, some new Medicare benefits, and some costs for clinical research studies.

- There is a monthly premium.
- There is an out-of-pocket maximum that once reached, results in no additional cost for Part A and B covered services.

To be eligible for a Medicare Advantage Plan, the enrollee must have Medicare Part A and Part B and live in the plan's service area.

Medicare Part D (Medicare Prescription Drug Coverage)

Medicare prescription drug coverage is an optional benefit that participants pay a premium for. To get Medicare prescription drug coverage, the participant must join a plan approved by Medicare that offers Medicare drug coverage. Each plan can vary in cost and specific drugs covered.

There are 2 ways to get Medicare prescription drug coverage:

1. Medicare Prescription Drug Plans. These plans (sometimes called "PDPs") add drug coverage to Original Medicare, some Medicare Cost Plans, some Medicare Private Fee-for-Service (PFFS) plans, and Medicare Medical Savings Account (MSA) plans. To be eligible the participant must have Medicare Part A and/or Part B.

2. Medicare Advantage Plans or other Medicare health plans that offer Medicare prescription drug coverage. Participants get all of their Part A, Part B, and prescription drug coverage (Part D), through these plans. Medicare Advantage Plans with prescription drug coverage are sometimes called "MA-PDs." The participant must have Part A and Part B to join a Medicare Advantage Plan, and not all of these plans offer drug coverage.

MEDIGAP

Original Medicare pays for much, but not all, of the cost for covered healthcare services and supplies. Medicare Supplemental Insurance policies are sold by private insurance companies to help cover Medicare's out-of-pocket expenses like copayments, coinsurance, and deductibles. Medicare Supplement Insurance policies are also called Medigap policies. Starting January 1, 2020,

Medigap plans sold to people who are new to Medicare won't be allowed to cover the Part B deductible.

To be eligible for a Medigap policy the enrollee must have Medicare Part A and Part B. Some Medigap policies also offer coverage for services that Original Medicare doesn't cover, like medical care when traveling outside the United States. Generally, Medigap policies don't cover long-term care, vision or dental care, hearing aids, eyeglasses, or private-duty nursing. (Medicare & You, 2020)

MEDICAID

Medicaid is a health insurance program funded jointly by the states and the federal government for individuals with limited income and resources. Medicaid also covers services not normally covered by Medicare, such as long-term support and services, as well as personal care services. According to the Centers for Medicare & Medicaid Services (2020), "Medicaid is the single largest source of health coverage in the United States."

To participate in Medicaid, federal law requires states to cover certain groups of individuals. Low-income families, qualified pregnant women and children, and individuals receiving Supplemental Security Income (SSI) are examples of mandatory eligibility groups. A complete list can be found at the link below.

https://www.medicaid.gov/sites/default/files/2019-12/list-of-eligibility-groups.pdf

States have additional options for coverage and may choose to cover other groups, such as individuals receiving home and community-based services and children in foster care who are not otherwise eligible.

The Affordable Care Act of 2010 created the opportunity for states to expand Medicaid to cover nearly all low-income Americans under age 65. Eligibility for children was extended to at least 133% of the federal poverty level (FPL) in every state (most states cover children to higher income levels), and states were given the option to extend eligibility to adults with income at or below 133% of the FPL.

Most states have chosen to expand coverage to adults, and those that have not yet expanded may choose to do so at any time.

States have the option to establish a "medically needy program" for individuals with significant health needs whose income is too high to otherwise qualify for Medicaid under other eligibility groups. Medically needy individuals can still become eligible by "spending down" the amount of income that is above a state's medically needy income standard. Individuals spend down by incurring expenses for medical and remedial care for which they do not have health insurance. Once an individual's incurred expenses exceed the difference between the individual's income and the state's medically needy income level (the "spend down" amount), the person can be eligible for Medicaid. The Medicaid program then pays the cost of services that exceeds the expenses the individual had to incur to become eligible.

To be eligible for Medicaid, individuals must also meet certain non-financial eligibility criteria. Medicaid beneficiaries generally must be residents of the state in which they are receiving Medicaid. They must be either citizens of the United States or certain qualified non-citizens, such as lawful permanent residents. In addition, some eligibility groups are limited by age, or by pregnancy or parenting status.

Once an individual is determined eligible for Medicaid, coverage is effective either on the date of application or the first day of the month of application. Benefits may also be covered retroactively up to three months prior to the month of application if the individual would have been eligible during the retroactive period. Coverage generally stops at the end of the month in which a person no longer meets the requirements for eligibility.

Medicaid Benefits

States establish and administer their Medicaid programs. They also determine the type, amount, duration, and scope of services, within the federal guidelines. States are required to cover certain "mandatory benefits" and can choose to provide "optional benefits." Generally speaking, Medicaid covers:

- Doctors visits
- Hospital stays
- Long-term services and supports (e.g., institutional care, home care, community-based long-term services)
- Preventive care, including immunizations, mammograms, and colonoscopies
- Prenatal and maternity care
- Mental health care
- Necessary medications
- Vision and dental care for children

Asset Considerations Related to Medicaid

Spousal Impoverishment: The expenses of nursing home care can rapidly deplete the savings of couples. In 1988 Congress enacted provisions to prevent what has come to be called "spousal impoverishment"—that is, when the spouse still living at home has little or no income or resources. Under the Medicaid spousal impoverishment provisions, a certain amount of the couple's combined resources is protected when one spouse needs coverage for long term services and supports (LTSS) in either an institution or a home or community-based setting, and is expected to remain there for at least 30 days.

Treatment of Trusts: When an individual, his or her spouse, or anyone acting on the individual's behalf establishes a trust using at least some of the individual's funds, that trust can be considered available to the individual for purposes of determining eligibility for Medicaid.

Transfers of Assets for Less Than Fair Market Value: Medicaid beneficiaries who need LTSS will be denied LTSS coverage if they have transferred assets for less than fair market value during the five-year period preceding their Medicaid application. This rule applies when individuals (or their spouses) who need LTSS in a long-term care facility or wish to receive home and community-based waiver services have transferred, sold, or gifted assets for less than they are worth.

Estate Recovery: State Medicaid programs must recover from a Medicaid enrollee's estate the cost of certain benefits paid on behalf of the enrollee. These benefits include nursing facilities services, home and community-based services, and related hospital and prescription drug services.

Medicaid Hospice Services

The Hospice benefit is an optional state plan service that includes an array of services furnished to terminally ill individuals. These services include:

- Nursing
- Medical social services
- Physician services
- Counseling services to the terminally ill individual and the family members or others caring for the individual at home
- Short-term inpatient care for pain control, symptom management, and respite care
- Medical equipment and supplies
- Home health aide and homemaker services
- Physical therapy
- Occupational therapy
- Speech-language pathology services
- Dietary counseling
- Medications for symptom control and pain relief

Medicaid pays a daily rate based on the level of care, same as Medicare does. Beginning March 23, 2010, with the enactment of the Affordable Care Act, Medicaid and Children's Health Insurance Program (CHIP) eligible individuals under age 21 who elect the hospice benefit no longer have to waive services for the cure or treatment of the terminal condition and can receive both curative care and hospice care for the terminal condition.

The eligibility requirements for hospice care under Medicaid are:

- Terminal illness certified by a physician

- Reduced life expectancy (stated by the physician) as defined by the state in which Medicaid is received
- Election of the hospice benefit
- Patient agrees to give up curative care in favor of care to manage symptoms and promote comfort unless the patient is younger than 21 years of age

SSDI

Social Security Disability Insurance, or SSDI, is an earned benefit, like the Social Security retirement benefit. It is given to those unable to work due to a physical or mental disability. To be eligible for SSDI, an individual must be unable to perform the work they previously did and not be able to adjust to other work because of the condition. The disability must be expected to last for at least one year or result in death. At age 65 the benefit automatically converts to the retirement benefit, but the benefit amount remains the same.

Overview of SSDI:

- Based on work record
- Funded by Social Security taxes paid by workers, employers, and the self-employed
- For those over age 18 and under 65
- Covers blind or disabled workers
- Focuses on physical and mental impairments severe enough to prevent engaging in normal occupation or any other work
- A 5-month waiting period for benefits to begin
- Approval for SSDI can come quickly if the individual has one of the serious medical conditions named on the Social Security Compassionate Allowance List; otherwise obtaining SSDI approval is a long process
- After receiving SSDI for 24 months, an individual is eligible for Medicare; including the 5-month waiting period, this equals 29 months before Medicare eligibility

- Like the Social Security retirement benefit, it can be paid to children, widows/widowers, and adults who haven't worked but have been disabled since childhood

SSI

Supplemental Security Income (SSI) is a need-based program that makes cash assistance payments to disabled individuals with limited income and resources. SSI is financed by general revenues collected by the Treasury Department. The disability criteria are the same as for SSDI. Individuals eligible for SSI are also eligible for Medicaid.

Benefit types:
- Age (65 and older) who meet the financial limits
- Disability (any age, includes children)
- Blindness (any age, includes children)

Comparison of Public Benefit Programs

	Medicare	Medicaid	SSDI	SSI
Benefit Type	Medical	Medical	Cash Benefit	Cash Benefit
Benefits based on	Earnings	Need	Earnings	Need
Financed by	Employer and wage contributions	General Revenues	Employer and wage contributions	General Revenues
Income/ Resource Limit for Eligibility	No limit	Income and resource limits	No limit	Income and resource limits
Work Credits Required	Yes	No	Yes	No
Basis for Benefit Amount	N/A	N/A	Average lifetime earnings	Federal and state laws

Military and Veteran Benefit Programs

TRICARE

TRICARE is the healthcare program for service members (active, Guard/Reserve, and retired) and their families. TRICARE is managed by the Defense Health Agency (DHA) and uses military healthcare as its main delivery system, supported by a civilian network of providers and facilities.

Who Is Eligible?

TRICARE is a health program for:
- Uniformed Service members and their families,
- National Guard/Reserve members and their families, which includes members of the:
    - Army National Guard
    - Army Reserve
    - Navy Reserve
    - Marine Corps Reserve
    - Air National Guard
    - Air Force Reserve
    - U.S. Coast Guard Reserve
- Survivors,
- Former spouses,
- Medal of Honor recipients and their families, and
- Others registered in the Defense Enrollment Eligibility Reporting System (DEERS).

The benefits and plans available will vary depending on the branch of the military, healthcare needs, and military activity status (active duty or retired) of the beneficiary. In general, TRICARE provides coverage for preventive care, vision and dental care, mental health, pharmacy services, and special programs for individuals with disabilities, in need of specialty treatments, or in different stages of duty—such as transitioning to careers outside the military sector. The healthcare services TRICARE covers vary among enrollees so it is important to look at the individual's plan.

TRICARE offers three basic options for care:
- TRICARE Prime: a managed care plan
- TRICARE Select: a fee-for-service plan
- TRICARE for Life: Medicare wraparound coverage for beneficiaries entitled to Medicare

TRICARE For Life

TRICARE For Life (TFL) is Medicare wraparound coverage for TRICARE beneficiaries who have Medicare Part A and Part B. It provides comprehensive healthcare coverage. Medicare is the primary payer. Beneficiaries can receive care from any Medicare participating or nonparticipating provider, as well as at any military clinic or hospital. If receiving services from a Medicare nonparticipating provider, TRICARE pays only the amount it would have paid if the beneficiary had gone to a Medicare participating provider (normally 20% of the TRICARE allowable charge).

VA

The Veterans Health Administration (VHA) is America's largest integrated healthcare system with over 1,255 sites of care, serving nine million veterans each year. Veterans of the United States Uniformed Services may be eligible for a broad range of programs and services provided by the Department of Veterans Affairs (VA).

VA Health Benefits include all the necessary inpatient hospital care and outpatient services to promote, preserve, or restore health. VHA medical facilities provide a wide range of services, including traditional hospital-based services such as surgery, critical care, mental health, orthopedics, pharmacy, radiology, and physical therapy.

Eligibility for most VA benefits is based upon discharge from active military service under other than dishonorable conditions. Many veterans qualify for cost-free healthcare based on a service-connected condition or other qualifying factors. Some veterans may be required to pay a copayment for treatment of their non-service-connected conditions.

Veterans can get free VA healthcare for any illness or injury that the VA determines is related to military service (called "service-connected"). The VA also provides certain other services for free. These include readjustment counseling and related mental health services, care for issues related to military sexual trauma (MST), and a registry health exam to determine the risk of health problems linked to military service. Veterans may qualify for additional free VA healthcare depending on their income, disability rating, or other special eligibility factors.

Veterans may need to pay a copayment for some types of care, tests, and medications they receive from a VA healthcare provider or an approved community healthcare provider to treat conditions not related to their service. Whether or not they will need to pay copayments and how much they will pay depends on their disability rating, income level, military service record, and which of the VA's eight priority groups they were assigned to when they enrolled in VA healthcare.

Tricare and VA Dual Eligibility

When leaving active duty, service members may be entitled to or eligible for benefits offered by TRICARE and the Department of Veterans Affairs (VA), depending on whether the service member retires or separates. If retiring, the service member is eligible for TRICARE as a military retiree and may also be eligible for certain VA benefits. Service members who separate due to a service-connected disease or disability may be eligible for VA benefits and certain TRICARE benefits.

If eligible, TRICARE provides coverage even if treatment is received through the VA for the same medical condition in a previous episode of care. However,

TRICARE will not duplicate payments made by the VA or authorized to be made by the VA. The rules and costs of whichever benefit is used will apply.

Reimbursement and Payment Methodologies

Until recently, providers and organizations have been paid based on a fee-for-service system. With fee-for-service reimbursement, each service rendered is priced separately. For example, mastectomy services would include charges for the hospital room, medications, surgical supplies, the OR suite, physician charges, surgeon charges, anesthesia, anesthesiologist, post-op office visits, and so on.

It is believed by some in the medical community that the fee-for-service payment system encourages the overuse of healthcare resources. To overcome this, several new reimbursement methods have been introduced in recent years. These include value-based reimbursement, financial risk models, and episode-of-care types of reimbursement.

Episode-of-care reimbursement models include bundled payments, case rates, and prospective payment systems. These reimbursement models attempt to correct the overuse of healthcare resources by paying one predetermined amount, no matter the number or cost of services provided.

Reimbursement and Payment methods at a glance:

Payment based on:
- Service provided
    - Fee-for-service
- Diagnosis or procedure (Average cost)
    - Bundled Payment
    - Case Rate
    - Prospective Payment

- Outcome
    - Value-based care
- Financial Risk
    - Shared Risk
    - Full Risk (capitation)

We will now look at each of these in detail.

Bundled/Case Rate

The terms bundled and case rate are used interchangeably, though there are some subtle differences. Both make a single payment for all services related to a treatment or condition. The term bundled is used more often when referring to "bundling" physician and hospital charges or charges to multiple providers in multiple settings. Case rate is used when referring to a flat fee paid to the provider for a client's treatment based on his diagnosis or presenting problem.

In general, both terms represent a single comprehensive payment made to healthcare providers to cover all of the services the client requires for a specific treatment or condition. Bundled or case rates are often used in orthopedic procedures such as total hip replacements, cardiac procedures such as CABG (coronary artery bypass grafting), and maternity care.

Prospective Payment System

A Prospective Payment System (PPS) is a method of reimbursement in which payment is made based on a predetermined, fixed amount. The PPS was developed to motivate providers to deliver patient care in a cost-effective, efficient manner without over-utilization of services. Providers know how much they will be reimbursed by the insurance company in advance and can either make money or lose money on the reimbursement. Where the traditional fee-for-service payment system can create an incentive to add unnecessary services, the PPS system discourages this.

The PPS also encourages efficiency. Where a hospital may have kept a patient over the weekend to perform a test or procedure on Monday, the PPS system incentivizes the hospital to call in staff to conduct it over the weekend. This can lead to faster diagnosis and treatment, shorter hospital stays, and ultimately lower costs.

Depending on the episode of care reimbursement agreement between the provider and the reimburser, once the initial admission is approved, continued stay review may not be necessary for patients admitted with procedures/diagnoses outlined in the PPS unless the patient has a large variance in the amount and/or level of care they are utilizing. This is because a predetermined reimbursement rate has been negotiated for all patients admitted with this diagnosis. If the patient is discharged early and/or utilizes fewer resources, the provider makes money. If the patient's discharge is delayed, the provider loses money.

Medicare's Prospective Payment System

Medicare's PPS determines the payment amount for a particular service based on the classification system of that service. For example, for an inpatient hospital stay, the classification system is the diagnosis-related group (DRG). Medicare uses separate payment systems for reimbursement to acute inpatient hospitals, home health agencies, hospice, hospital outpatient, inpatient psychiatric facilities, inpatient rehabilitation facilities, long-term care hospitals, and skilled nursing facilities.

For acute inpatient hospitals, the inpatient prospective payment system (IPPS) is used. Under the IPPS, each case is categorized into a DRG. Each DRG has a payment weight assigned to it, based on the average resources used to treat Medicare patients in that DRG.

Other Medicare Prospective Payment Systems

Inpatient Rehabilitation Facilities

When a patient enters an inpatient rehabilitation hospital they are assessed with the Inpatient Rehabilitation Facilities Patient Assessment Instrument (IRF-PAI). This is used to classify the patient into a distinct group based on clinical characteristics and expected resource needs. The PAI determines the Case Mix Group (CMG) classification which determines the payment rate for this stay.

Outpatient Hospital

Outpatient hospitals including hospital-based clinics, emergency departments, observation, and ambulatory surgery centers use the Ambulatory Payment Classification System (APC). This is an encounter based classification system for outpatient reimbursement. Payment rates are based on categories of services that are similar in cost and resource utilization.

Home Health Agencies and Skilled Nursing Facilities

As part of overall efforts to move Medicare payment away from fee-for-service and toward a structure that holds providers accountable for patient outcomes and costs, the Centers for Medicare and Medicaid Services (CMS) has made significant changes to the home health and skilled nursing facility (SNF) payment systems. Both of these payment systems align payment with patient characteristics, conditions, and needs, and eliminate the connection between reimbursement and the volume of therapy services provided—time spent and number of visits. Under both models, ICD-10 codes form the basis of reimbursement.

Home Health

Upon admission to home health, the patient is assessed using the Outcome and Assessment Information Set (OASIS). This is a prospective nursing assessment instrument that's score, along with other data on the patient, determines the Home Health Resource Group (HHRG) the patient will be placed in. The HHRG sets the reimbursement rate.

CMS finalized a new case-mix classification model, the Patient-Driven Groupings Model (PDGM), effective beginning January 1, 2020. The PDGM relies more heavily on clinical characteristics and other patient information to place home health periods of care into meaningful payment categories. One case-mix variable is the assignment of the principal diagnosis to one of 12 clinical groups to explain the primary reason for home health services. Payment is based on this assignment.

Skilled Nursing Facilities

CMS finalized a new case-mix classification model, the Patient Driven Payment Model (PDPM), effective beginning October 1, 2019. The PDPM is used under the Skilled Nursing Facility (SNF) Prospective Payment System (PPS) for classifying SNF patients in a covered Part A stay.

Value-Based Care

Value-based care agreements are designed to reward providers, including hospitals and physicians, for helping patients to improve their health, reduce the negative effects of chronic disease, and live healthier lives in an evidence-based way. Value-based care aims to accomplish this by linking payment to patient health outcomes. Providers who provide higher value care will receive higher payments than those who provide lower-quality care.

The Affordable Care Act established the Hospital Value-Based Purchasing (VBP) Program. VBP is a CMS initiative that rewards acute-care hospitals with incentive payments for the quality of care they provide to Medicare beneficiaries. CMS bases hospital performance on an approved set of measures and dimensions grouped into specific quality domains. These domains vary depending on the program's fiscal year. VBP uses quality measures that hospitals already report to Medicare via the Hospital Inpatient Quality Reporting program.

Case managers play a critical role in helping move to a value-based system. They improve outcomes by developing a patient-centered plan of care, facilitating transitions of care, and improving communication between the interprofessional team.

Financial Risk Models

Financial risk models of reimbursement are used by HMOs and aim to control costs and prevent the overutilization of resources by having the provider take on some, or all, of the financial responsibility for their members' care.

Two common financial risk models are risk sharing and capitation. With risk sharing, the HMO and contracted provider each accept partial responsibility for the financial risk and rewards involved in cost-effectively caring for the members enrolled in the plan and assigned to the provider. With capitation, the provider or provider organization(s) take on more risk because they agree to receive a set payment per-member-per-month(PMPM) for specified medical services from the payer.

Population Health

With reimbursement shifting from volume to value, providers are seeking ways to improve the health and wellness of the population they serve. Population health management is a crucial component for healthcare providers to improve care quality and lower costs. The goal is to improve the health of a given geographical area, improve the delivery of care, and contain healthcare costs.

To accomplish this, population health focuses on prevention and disease management by:
- Identifying high-risk, high-cost patients
- Preventing or minimizing the progression of disease(s)
- Promoting a culture of wellness

This requires an interdisciplinary, customizable approach. Each population served has a unique set of obstacles to overcome and strengths to pull from.

A successful population health program will bring significant health concerns of the population served into focus, and address ways that resources can be allocated to overcome the problems that drive poor health conditions in that population.

Coding Methodologies

Medical coding is the transformation of healthcare diagnoses, procedures, and medical services into universal medical alphanumeric codes. The codes are used by healthcare providers, government health programs, health insurance companies, and others. Uses include:

- Reimbursement (filing and processing claims)
- Tracking infectious diseases (such as the flu, TB, and whooping cough)
- Tracking health conditions (such as diabetes, cardiovascular disease, and cancer)

International Classification of Diseases (ICD)

The International Classification of Diseases (ICD) coding system assigns a number or alphanumeric to describe diseases, traumas, and environmental circumstances leading to bodily harm. It is used to report medical diagnoses and procedures on claims as well as to gain data for public health surveillance. The code set, which was updated to ICD-10 in 2015, consists of two parts:

- ICD-10-CM – (Clinical Modification) The diagnosis classification system used by all healthcare providers.
- ICD-10-PCS – (Procedure Coding System) The procedure classification system used for inpatient procedure reporting in hospitals.

The ICD code is the diagnosis/reason for the encounter with the health system (e.g., chest pain, pre-op evaluation, diabetes).

Current Procedural Terminology (CPT)

Current Procedural Terminology (CPT) codes are maintained and copyrighted by the American Medical Association (AMA). They are a standardized form of identifying services provided, including medical, surgical, radiology, laboratory, anesthesiology, and evaluation and management services. Providers use CPT codes to report services performed to payers for reimbursement purposes, assigning a code for each procedure done during that visit. While the ICD-10 code tells the reason for the visit (e.g., chest pain), the CPT code lists the procedures performed (e.g., evaluation and management, venipuncture, ECG).

Diagnosis Related Group (DRG)

Medicare uses the Diagnosis Related Group (DRG) system as a basis of payment for hospital inpatient services. In an attempt to control costs, hospitals are paid based on the DRG for the admission rather than for each procedure performed or inpatient day.

DRG combines ICD-10 codes with patient demographics, discharge status, and the presence of complications or comorbidities to classify a hospital admission into a payment category, based on the assumption that similar diagnoses should have similar hospital resource use and length of stay patterns.

The ICD-10 is used in determining the DRG, and the DRG is used to determine reimbursement for Medicare and some other payers.

Diagnostic and Statistical Manual of Mental Disorders (DSM)

The Diagnostic and Statistical Manual of Mental Disorders (DSM) is the official classification and listing of mental disorders. It contains descriptions, symptoms, and other criteria for diagnosing mental disorders. It provides a common language for clinicians to communicate about their patients and establishes consistent and reliable diagnoses.

Each diagnosis includes a diagnostic code that providers, institutions, and agencies use for billing and data collection. The newest in the series, the

DSM-5, includes both the older ICD-9 code related to the disorder, as well as the updated ICD-10 code in parentheses. There may be multiple disorders associated with a given ICD code; for this reason, it is recommended that the disorder be entered in the medical record by name as well as the code.

Accountable Care Organization

The Affordable Care Act authorized the Center for Medicare and Medicaid Services (CMS) to create the Medicare Shared Savings program, which allows for the establishment of ACO contracts with Medicare.

A Medicare ACO is formed by a group of doctors, hospitals, and other healthcare providers that come together voluntarily to give coordinated, high-quality care to the Medicare Fee-for-Service beneficiaries they serve. Providers in ACOs are held jointly accountable for delivering care more efficiently by achieving reductions in the rate of spending growth and measured quality improvements (measured using ACO Quality Measures). They become eligible for bonuses when this is accomplished.

The goal of an ACO is to deliver seamless, high-quality care for Medicare beneficiaries, in contrast to the fragmented care that has so often been characteristic of fee-for-service healthcare. By providing coordinated care, patients get the right care at the right time, while avoiding unnecessary duplication of services and preventing medical errors. The ACO is a patient-centered organization, where the patient and providers are partners in care decisions.

When an ACO succeeds in the dual goals of delivering high-quality care and spending healthcare dollars more wisely, it shares in the savings it achieves for the Medicare program. This incentivizes the ACO to improve the coordination and quality of care for all its patients.

Core components of the ACO model of care are:

- Provider-led, with a strong base in primary care
- All providers, across the full continuum of care, are accountable for quality and cost related to a population of patients
- Payments are linked to quality improvements that reduce overall costs
- Performance is measured

Models of Care

Patient Centered Medical Home (PCMH)

The Patient-Centered Medical Home provides comprehensive primary care for children, youth, and adults. This healthcare setting facilitates long-term partnerships between patients, their personal physicians, and when appropriate, patients' families. Healthcare workers advocate for their patients and provide the education and support patients need to participate in and make decisions for their own care. The goal is to attain optimal, patient-centered outcomes that respect patients' wants, needs, and preferences. Unlike the ACO, the PCMH is a single practice.

Principles of the Patient-Centered Medical Home:

- Personal physician – Each patient has an ongoing relationship with a personal physician trained to provide first contact, continuous, and comprehensive care. This personal physician coordinates all care for the patient.
- Physician-directed medical practice – The personal physician leads a team of practicing healthcare providers who are collectively responsible for the ongoing care of the patient.
- Whole person orientation – The personal physician is responsible for providing for the patient's entire healthcare needs or appropriately arranging care with other qualified professionals. This includes care for all stages of life, acute care, chronic care, preventive services, and end of life care.

- Care is coordinated and/or integrated across all elements of the complex healthcare system (e.g., subspecialty care, hospitals, home health agencies, nursing homes) and the patient's community (e.g., family, public and private community-based services). Care is facilitated by registries, information technology, health information exchange, and other means. This ensures that patients get required care when and where they need and want it, in a culturally and linguistically appropriate manner.

- Enhanced access to care is available through systems such as open scheduling, expanded hours, and new options for communication between patients, their personal physicians, and practice staff.

- Evidence-based medicine and clinical decision-support tools guide decision- making.

- Physicians accept accountability for continuous quality improvement through voluntary engagement in performance measurement and improvement.

- The patient's participation in decision-making and feedback is sought to ensure his expectations are being met.

- Information technology is utilized appropriately to support optimal patient care, performance measurement, patient education, and enhanced communication.

Health Home

Healthcare for individuals with multiple chronic conditions comprises our nation's most costly and complex cases. According to the National Comorbidity Survey, of individuals with a mental illness, 68% also have a physical health condition such as cardiovascular disease, diabetes, or hypertension. These high-need individuals often receive uncoordinated care that results in higher costs and poorer health outcomes.

Healthcare reform legislation established health homes as a new state Medicaid option for service delivery specifically for enrollees with chronic conditions.

A Medicaid health home, as defined in Section 2703 of the Affordable Care Act, offers coordinated care to individuals with multiple chronic health conditions, including mental health and substance use disorders. The health home recognizes the importance of caring for the whole person.

The health home is a team-based clinical approach that includes the consumer, his providers, and family members, when appropriate. The health home builds linkages to community support and resources, as well as enhances coordination and integration of primary and behavioral healthcare to better meet the needs of people with multiple chronic illnesses. The model aims to improve healthcare quality while also reducing costs. Health Home services include:

- Comprehensive care management
- Care coordination and health promotion
- Comprehensive transitional care from inpatient to other settings
- Individual family support
- Referral to community and social support services
- Use of health information technology to link services

Health home services are available to adults and children who receive benefits from Medicaid and who have at least two chronic conditions, such as asthma, diabetes, heart disease, obesity, a mental health condition, or substance abuse disorder; one chronic condition and are at risk for another; or one serious and persistent mental health condition.

Federal health home guidance lays out service requirements emerging from the ACA. The required services (also termed "provider standards" in the guidance) include:

- Each patient must have a comprehensive care plan
- Services must be quality-driven, cost-effective, culturally appropriate, person- and family-centered, and evidence-based
- Services must include prevention and health promotion, healthcare, mental health and substance use, and long-term care services, as well as linkages to community supports and resources

- Service delivery must involve continuing care strategies, including care management, care coordination, and transitional care from the hospital to the community
- Health home providers do not need to provide all the required services themselves but must ensure the full array of services is available and coordinated
- Providers must be able to use health information technology (HIT) to facilitate the health home's work and establish quality improvement efforts to ensure that the work is effective at the individual and population level

What is the difference between a medical home and a health home?

	Medical Homes	Health Homes
Population Served	Serve all populations	Serve individuals with approved chronic conditions
Providers	Typically defined as physician-led primary care practices, but also mid-level practitioners and health centers	May include primary care practices, community mental health centers, federally qualified health centers, health home agencies, etc.
Payer(s)	Multiple payers (e.g., Medicare, Medicaid, commercial insurance)	Medicaid only
Care Focus	Focus on the delivery of traditional medical care (referral and lab tracking, guideline adherence, electronic prescribing, provider-patient communication)	Strong focus on whole health (including substance abuse, mental health, and primary care), social support, and other services (such as nutrition, home health, and coordinating activities)
Use of IT	For traditional care delivery	For coordination across continuum of care, including in-home (e.g., wireless monitoring)

Chronic Care Model

The Chronic Care Model is a method of caring for people with chronic disease in the primary care setting. It encourages practical, supportive, and evidence-based chronic disease management using a proactive (rather than responsive) approach. This approach results in patients who take an active part in their care. The Chronic Care Model has led to improved patient care and better outcomes for patients with chronic illness.

Six Components to the Chronic Care Model

1. Health System – This component addresses the culture, leadership, and practices of the organization, which encourages optimal management of chronic disease.

2. Delivery System – The delivery system provides efficient clinical care and self-management support. Rather than reactively treating the patient in crisis, the focus is on keeping the patient healthy and out of a crisis by providing follow-up care after the patient leaves the doctor's office. For more complex patients, case management is provided.

3. Self Management Support – This component focuses on empowering patients to manage their healthcare. Providers and patients use a collaborative approach to identify problems, set priorities and goals, create treatment plans, and solve problems.

4. Decision Support – Treatment is determined by discussing evidence-based guidelines with the patient so he or she becomes a participant in the decision- making process. Providers must keep up to date on the latest evidence and involve specialists when appropriate.

5. Clinical Information Systems – This component focuses on the organization of patient data to ensure the efficient and successful management of chronic disease.

6. Community Resources – Resources available in the community for care, peer support, and education expand on the health system's treatment of chronic illness.

Healthcare Delivery Systems

A healthcare delivery system is a combination of organizations and individuals that work together to provide healthcare to individuals. They can be public or private sector, including for-profit and not-for-profit. Examples include the military medical care system, and integrated delivery systems, as well as managed care delivery systems which include Health Maintenance Organizations (HMOs), Preferred Provider Organizations (PPOs), Point of Service Plans (POSs), and Exclusive Provider Organizations (EPOs).

Managed Care

Managed care organizations provide healthcare to members using contracted providers. These providers may include physicians, hospitals, nursing homes, medical equipment suppliers, and diagnostic clinics. They agree to provide care at a discounted rate to members. You will learn more about managed care in the sections on Cost Containment Principles and Managed Care Concepts.

Integrated Delivery System

CCMC in their Glossary of Terms defines an integrated delivery system as a single organization or group of affiliated organizations that provide a wide spectrum of ambulatory and tertiary care and services. Care may also be provided across various settings of the healthcare continuum.

An integrated delivery system is a variety of providers and/or organizations that come together to provide a coordinated continuum of services to a defined population. It could join physicians groups and hospitals, as is the case with a Physician Hospital Organization, or an insurance company with hospital and physician groups. If the integrated delivery system includes an insurance company, the physicians and hospitals are owned by or partner with the insurance company, rather than contracted by the insurance company (as with managed care organizations). The goal is to coordinate the seamless delivery of healthcare services.

Cost Containment Principles

Traditional Insurance Cost Containment

With traditional insurance, cost containment comes in the form of coinsurance, copayments, and deductibles.

A copayment is a set amount the patient pays each time a specific service is rendered. For example, a plan may require a $20 copayment for each doctor's office visit, or a $15 copayment for a prescription refill. Each time a patient goes to the doctor or has a prescription refilled, he will be charged the copayment amount, regardless of whether his deductible has been met.

The deductible and coinsurance work together. The deductible is a specific amount of money the patient must pay for covered expenses before the insurance company begins paying. Once the deductible has been paid, the coinsurance kicks in, with the insurance company and the patient sharing the remaining costs until maximum out of pocket limit is reached.

To illustrate: A patient received a procedure costing $5,000 and his plan required a $500 deductible and 80/20 coinsurance. The patient is first responsible for the $500 deductible. After that, the insurance company pays 80% of the remaining $4,500 (equaling $3,600), and the patient pays 20% coinsurance (equaling $900). The patient is responsible for $1,400 in total: the $500 deductible and the $900 coinsurance.

Managed Care Cost Containment

In managed care, medical services are coordinated by the insurance company to decrease healthcare costs. The two main types of managed care organizations are Preferred Provider Organizations (PPOs) and Health Maintenance Organizations (HMOs).

The PPO contains costs by negotiating discounts for services with providers as a condition for being included in the PPO. By receiving a discount from providers, the PPO is able to reduce health insurance premiums and healthcare expenditures. In turn, patients' costs are covered by the insurance company at a higher percentage when they choose providers in the PPO. Patients may choose providers not included in the PPO but will pay more out of pocket.

HMOs provide healthcare services to members for a set yearly fee per member. Providing too much or too costly care could cause them to lose money. Preventive care is encouraged under this insurance structure, to avoid more costly corrective care. HMOs often use a Primary Care Provider (PCP) to act as a gatekeeper. The gatekeeper's role is to provide medical and preventive care and to coordinate patient care outside of their scope of practice.

Medicare and DRG Cost Containment

Medicare implemented the diagnosis related group (DRG) system, in which the DRG pays a fixed amount for a given diagnosis, rather than paying all costs related to an individual patient's treatment during his hospital stay. This predetermined amount is paid regardless of the actual cost of treating the patient. This approach provides a significant incentive for hospitals to decrease costs.

Managed Care Concepts

Managed care is a system of healthcare delivery whose goal is to maintain quality, cost-efficient care by managing the use, access, cost, quality, and effectiveness of services. Managed care organizations link the patient to the provider and/or service and include several types, such as a preferred provider organization (PPO), exclusive provider organization (EPO), point-of-service (POS) plan, and health maintenance organization (HMO).

PPO

PPOs contract with providers of medical care to deliver care at a discounted rate. The providers with whom they contract are considered "preferred providers" or "network providers."

PPOs encourage the use of these preferred providers by providing significantly better benefits for services received by them. If the patient uses a provider who is not part of the network, he will incur greater financial responsibility for the healthcare services received.

EPO

An EPO is similar to a PPO in that a network of providers have agreed to provide care for the members at a discounted rate. In an EPO, however, a patient is not reimbursed for services if he chooses to receive healthcare outside the network.

Point-of-Service (POS)

The Point-of-Service Plan allows the patient to choose to receive care in-network at little or no cost or to go out of the network and incur larger out-of-pocket expenses.

HMO

HMOs reimburse providers by capitation, paying a fixed amount per-member-per-month for contracted services. Providers are not reimbursed for the specific services provided. If the member uses the services once, or more often, the provider receives the same payment. Services that are not included in the contract between the provider and the HMO can be "carve out" services. They are handled by other providers without penalty to the primary care physician (PCP). This is usually done for specialty services, such as transplant or mental/behavioral health.

HMOs often use the primary care physician as a "gatekeeper." A patient receives all primary and preventive care from the PCP, and any care needed that falls outside the PCP's scope of practice is referred out and coordinated by the PCP. Any care (other than emergency care) not coordinated through the PCP is not covered by the HMO.

There are four types of HMOs:

- Group Model HMO
- Network Model HMO
- Individual Practice Association (IPA) Model HMO
- Staff Model HMO

In the Group Model HMO, the HMO contracts with a multi-specialty physician group, where the physicians are employed by the group, not the HMO. The HMO and the group share profits or losses.

The Network Model HMO is similar to the group model but involves more than one group of physicians. In this model the HMO contracts with multiple groups of physicians and other providers to form a network of care. Networks allow providers to practice outside of the HMO.

The Individual Practice Association Model HMO contracts with physicians who provide healthcare to the HMO members for a negotiated rate. The physicians own their individual or group practices.

In the Staff Model, HMO physicians are employed by the HMO and provide services exclusively to members of the HMO.

Under the Federal HMO Act, an organization must possess the following to call itself an HMO:

1. An organized system for providing healthcare in a geographic area

2. An agreed on set of basic and supplemental health maintenance and treatment services

3. A voluntarily enrolled group of people

Utilization Management Principles and Guidelines

Utilization management ensures that services provided are at or above quality standards, provided at the appropriate and least costly level of care, and are medically necessary. Determining medical necessity for a procedure or level of service is often subjective resulting in inconsistency with approvals and denials. For this reason, many organizations use software such as MCG or InterQual to assist with utilization management. These tools were created using research and evidence-based guidelines, making the process more objective and establishing consistency. It is important to remember that these are only guidelines and that the expert opinion of the nurse, physician, or other healthcare professional is an important component in determining medical necessity.

**See Factors Used to Identify Acuity or Severity Levels for more information on MCG and InterQual.

The Utilization Review Process

1. Verify eligibility; that is, check that the patient is covered under the health plan and that this coverage is primary. For example: The patient may have both Medicare and insurance through his employer. The preauthorization request would go through the primary insurance first.

2. Verify that the requested service is a covered benefit under the insurance contract. If it is a covered benefit, determine if it requires preauthorization. For example, bariatric surgery may be a contract exclusion. If it is a covered benefit, it may require preauthorization.

3. Gather clinical information to determine if the criteria are met for this service.

4. Review clinical information to determine if it meets criteria for medical necessity and level of care, documenting as per policy.

5. If guidelines are met, notify the requesting provider of the approval.

6. If guidelines are not met, it is sent for physician review. The physician will approve or deny it based on medical judgment, and the requesting provider is notified of the decision.

7. If it is denied, the patient or treating physician may appeal.

8. The medical director collects more information and reviews the case again. They may also speak with the treating physician or send the information to an independent third party physician with expertise in the specialty area of the request.

There are three main types of utilization management: prospective, concurrent, and retrospective.

Prospective reviews, or precertifications, are done prior to the elective admission or procedure to ensure the requested service is necessary, meets criteria for coverage, and is at the appropriate level of care.

Concurrent reviews include continued stay reviews and are conducted as the care is occurring. This includes reviews for admissions that were not precertified, as well as to extend care that was precertified. Concurrent reviews are done to ensure the client is receiving the correct care in a timely and cost-effective manner.

The *retrospective review* is done after care has already occurred. This can occur when precertification was required but not obtained, such as in an emergency situation.

Factors Used to Identify Client's Acuity or Severity Levels

The diagnosis is only one factor in evaluating the acuity level of the patient. Other factors that may be taken into account include:

- Comorbid conditions
- Intensity of intervention needed
- Complex medical needs
- Family/social support
- Polypharmacy
- Psychological/cognitive status
- Complex treatment plans
- Number of providers involved

Acuity or severity levels are used for staffing as well as ensuring that the client is receiving the correct level of service. Two tools used to ensure the client is receiving the correct level of service are MCG Health and InterQual.

MCG Health provides evidence-based care solutions spanning the continuum of care, including:

- Ambulatory Care
- Inpatient & Surgical Care

- General Recovery Care
- Recovery Facility Care
- Home Care
- Behavioral Health Care

InterQual Level of Care Criteria helps healthcare organizations assess the clinical appropriateness of patient services across the continuum of care. The severity of illness, comorbidities, and complications, as well as the intensity of services being delivered, guide them to the most efficient and safest level of care.

InterQual Level of Care Criteria are available for:
- Acute Care
- Acute Pediatric
- Acute Rehabilitation
- Long-Term Acute Care
- Subacute Care and Skilled Nursing Facility
- Home Care
- Outpatient Rehabilitation and Chiropractic

Levels of Care and Care Settings

Acute Care

Acute care is the most intensive level of care, during which a patient is treated for a brief but severe episode of illness, for conditions that are the result of disease or trauma, and/or during recovery from surgery. Acute care is generally provided in a hospital by a physician and a variety of clinical personnel.

Long-Term Acute Care Hospitals and Long-Term Care Hospitals

According to Centers for Medicare & Medicaid Services (CMS), long-term acute care hospitals (LTAC)—also referred to as long-term care hospitals (LTCH) and transitional hospitals—focus on patients whose length of stay is greater than 25 days on average. Many of the patients in LTACs are transferred in from an intensive or critical care unit. LTACs specialize in treating patients who have one or more serious conditions but who may improve with time and care. Services provided in LTACs typically include comprehensive rehabilitation, respiratory therapy, head trauma treatment, and pain management.

Subacute Care

Subacute care is for patients who are stable and do not require hospital acute care, but who require more intensive skilled nursing care, therapy, and physician services than are provided to the majority of patients in a skilled nursing facility. These services may include TPN, IV therapy, wound care, and other therapies such as speech therapy, physical therapy, occupational therapy, and respiratory therapy.

Inpatient Rehabilitation

Inpatient rehabilitation hospitals provide intense, multidisciplinary therapy to patients with a functional loss. To qualify for this level of care, patients must be able to tolerate a minimum of three hours of therapy per day, five to seven days per week, and be medically stable.

Skilled Nursing Facility (SNF)

SNFs offer 24-hour skilled nursing and personal care (e.g., bathing, eating, toileting). They also provide rehabilitation services, such as physical therapy, occupational therapy, and speech therapy. Patients must be medically stable to qualify for SNF level of care. They also must need care from a skilled, licensed professional, such as a nurse or therapist, on a daily basis. Examples are complex wound care and rehabilitation when a patient cannot tolerate three hours of therapy per day.

Intermediate Care

Intermediate care is a level of care for patients who require more assistance than custodial care and may require nursing supervision, but do not have a true skilled need. Most insurance companies do not cover intermediate care.

Home Health Care

Home health care provides intermittent skilled care to patients in their home. Services such as skilled nursing, physical therapy, occupational therapy, speech therapy, and medical social worker visits are provided by home health agencies. For a patient to qualify for home health care under Medicare, he must be deemed homebound. To qualify as homebound, the patient must be unable to leave his home or requires great effort to leave.

Hospice Care

Hospice provides end of life care to patients with a terminal illness. It also supports their families. To qualify for hospice care, a physician must document that the patient's life expectancy is limited if the disease follows its normal course of progression. Hospice care can be provided in any setting, including the patient's home, in the hospital, in a skilled nursing facility, or in a freestanding hospice facility.

Custodial Care

Custodial care assists with personal and home care, such as ADLs (activities of daily living) and IADLs (instrumental activities of daily living). This level does not require the services of a skilled or licensed provider. Custodial care can take place in the home, a skilled nursing facility, or an assisted living facility, among other places. Medical insurance does not cover this level of care.

Alternative Care Facilities

Assisted Living

Assisted living facilities provide housing and support with ADLs and IADLs to residents. Services provided often include:

- Meals
- Medication reminders

- Transportation
- Housekeeping
- Laundry
- 24-hour staff
- Personal assistance with ADLs

Assisted living facilities do not provide medical care or skilled nursing care. The cost of assisted living is not covered by medical insurance; it is paid either by the individual and his family or, if purchased, a long-term care insurance policy. Medicaid waiver programs may also cover assisted living. States, not the federal government, regulate these types of facilities.

Group Homes

Residents of group homes are typically children or adults with chronic disabilities requiring continual assistance to complete ADLs/IADLs or behavioral problems that make them dangerous to themselves or others. Group homes usually house fewer than eight residents who share common areas such as the kitchen, living room, and laundry facilities and are staffed by trained personnel. The residents, depending on their ability, do chores.

Residential Treatment Facilities

Residential treatment facilities house and provide therapy for patients with drug and alcohol addictions, emotional or behavioral problems, and/or mental illness. They are clinically focused and offer treatments such as psychoanalytic therapy, behavioral management, group counseling, family therapy, and medication management. Residents have usually been unsuccessful with outpatient treatments, but are not appropriate for an inpatient psychiatric unit.

Alternative Care Sites (e.g., non-traditional sites of care, telehealth, virtual care)

The use of technology, such as the telephone, audio and/or video equipment, or the internet to provide healthcare is becoming more common. These technologies provide a new setting of care: virtual care. Virtual care allows the case manager to deliver efficient and effective professional case management services to a greater number of clients than face-to-face care. It also allows case managers and other providers to reach clients that are in rural or remote areas where access to providers is a challenge.

Assessment, care coordination, education, and management of services can all be done virtually, but to be effective in this alternative care setting, there are some things that will need to be considered. Case managers must be extremely competent in assessment, critical thinking, communication, and problem-solving to be successful in the virtual setting. They also need to be able to practice independently while cooperating with other team members that may not be on site.

Another important consideration is licensure. Case managers must be licensed in the state where case management is being provided. Telephonic case managers who manage cases across state lines must be licensed in the state where the client is located. The Nurse Licensure Compact gives nurses the ability to practice nursing across state lines. The nurse must be licensed in her state of residency. If the state of residency participates in the compact, she can practice in any other compact state.

Compliance with the Health Insurance Portability and Accountability Act (HIPAA) is another important consideration in virtual care. HIPAA guidelines on telemedicine are contained within the HIPAA Security Rule and require a system of secure communication be implemented to protect the integrity of electronic protected health information (ePHI). This means that unsecured methods of communication such as text, Skype, and email can not be used "as is" and will need to be secured to be used. Organizations that use telehealth and virtual care will have acceptable means of communication in their policies and procedures to ensure secure message transmission.

Need Additional Support?

This chapter contained a lot of heavy information and can be difficult to get through, but is important to understand. If you are someone who learns best by hearing the information in a more conversational style or needs accountability to stay motivated, we have additional resources for you. We offer 2 CCM Prep Courses to meet your individual needs. You can find more information at

CCMcertificationMadeEasy.com

References

Centers for Medicare & Medicaid Services. (n.d.). https://www.cms.gov/

Centers for Medicare & Medicaid Services. (n.d.). *Eligibility*. https://www.medicaid.gov/medicaid/eligibility/index.html

Centers for Medicare & Medicaid Services. (2019, December). *Medicare & you*. https://www.medicare.gov/Pubs/pdf/10050-Medicare-and-You.pdf

Commission for Case Management Certification. (2017). *Glossary of terms*. https://ccmcertification.org/get-certified/exam-study-materials/ccmc-glossary

Employee Benefits Security Administration. (2018, September). *An employer's guide to group health continuation coverage under COBRA*. https://www.dol.gov/sites/dolgov/files/EBSA/about-ebsa/our-activities/resource-center/publications/an-employers-guide-to-group-health-continuation-coverage-under-cobra.pdf

Kessler, R.C. (1990-1992 Restricted Version). National Comorbidity Survey: Baseline (NCS-1). Inter-University Consortium for Political and Social Research, 2009.

National Association of Insurance Commissioners. (2013). *Coordination of benefits model regulation*. https://www.naic.org/store/free/MDL-120.pdf

<<<< >>>>

Test Your Knowledge On Care Delivery and Reimbursement Methods

1. Which case management step involves reviewing information to decide a patient's appropriateness for case management services?

    A. Case planning

    B. Assessment

    C. Stratifying risk

    D. Screening

2. Which important activity should be included during the transitioning step of the case management process?

    A. Assessing whether the client is ready for transfer to another level of care

    B. Assessing the effectiveness of the case management plan

    C. Assessing the patient's knowledge of their health conditions

    D. Assessing the patient's belief in self-efficacy

3. Which assessment tool evaluates areas of function for self-care?

    A. Activities of Daily Living

    B. Behavioral Assessment

    C. Patient Health Questionnaire

    D. Health Risk Assessments

4. What assessment tool is used to pre-screen patients for depression?

    A. PHQ-9

    B. Instrumental Activities of Daily living

    C. PHQ-2

    D. Wellness screenings

5. Case manager Mary is preparing to move her patient from an acute hospital setting to a skilled nursing facility. What should Mary keep in mind during this transition of care?

   A. Her patient needs to understand the reason for moving to another level of care.

   B. Her patient needs to have all their medications with them.

   C. Her patient is at increased risk for adverse outcomes.

   D. Her patient needs to be educated on self-management.

6. What best describes the role of an Interdisciplinary team?

   A. Work in a group to manage a patient's transition of care

   B. Work in a group to develop policies and processes of patient care

   C. Work in a group to review adverse events of care

   D. Work in a group to manage the physical, psychological, and spiritual needs of the patient

7. Hospice care provides:

   A. End of life care for only Medicare patients with a terminal illness

   B. End of life care, including palliative care, to patients with a terminal illness

   C. End of life care that excludes palliative care to patients with a terminal illness

   D. End of life care for only Medicaid patients with a terminal illness

8. Which statement about Social Security Disability Income (SSDI) is true?

   A. It is a needs-based benefit

   B. There is no waiting period

   C. It is funded by Social Security taxes paid by workers and employers

D. Eligibility is based on income

9. Coordination of benefits is designed to:

A. Maximize benefits to patients

B. Provide a reimbursement methodology when there is more than one payment source

C. Provide a replacement for lost wages as well as medical coverage

D. Assure the contractual requirements for coverage are met

10. Which of the following is not a payment methodology?

A. Fee for service

B. Prospective payment

C. Accountable care

D. Bundled case rate

11. Selling a life insurance policy to a third party for cash is called a:

A. Reverse mortgage

B. Viatical settlement

C. Actuarial calculation

D. Accelerated death benefit

12. Medicare Part D covers:

A. Home care

B. Inpatient rehab

C. Prescription medications

D. Outpatient PT/OT

13. Precertification is:

    A. The process of applying for health insurance

    B. The required amount of time one must work before becoming eligible for coverage.

    C. The waiting period for disability

    D. The process of obtaining approval before medical treatment occurs

14. What form of coverage does not have a waiting period?

    A. Short term disability insurance

    B. Long term disability insurance

    C. Workers' compensation

    D. Social Security Disability

15. Medicare Part A will cover a patient in a skilled nursing facility if:

    A. Their PCP orders the stay and it is medically necessary

    B. It is medically necessary and immediately follows a hospital stay of at least one week

    C. The patient lives alone and can't care for himself

    D. It follows within 30 days of a hospital stay of at least 3 days and is medically necessary

16. A patient in an Exclusive Provider Organization (EPO) plan decides to go out-of-network to receive care. This decision means that he will:

    A. Be subject to a large deductible and copay

    B. Not be covered under the health plan for the services provided

    C. Will be covered

    D. Be converted to a fee-for-services plan

17. The insurance case manager requests information from the hospital case manager about a patient's current status including labs, vitals, and wound healing. This is:

   A. A retrospective review

   B. A concurrent review

   C. A peer to peer review

   D. A prospective review

18. A copayment is a:

   A. Specific amount paid at the time of the service for specified services

   B. Your monthly premium

   C. The amount of the premium paid after your employer contributes

   D. The amount you must pay before your insurance begins paying

19. The case management process includes:

   A. Assessing, planning, implementing, coordinating, monitoring, and evaluating

   B. Quality Improvement, analysis, and monitoring

   C. Contacting the client, validating insurance, coordinating care, and billing

   D. Assessing, diagnosing, coordinating, and utilization management

20. An Accelerated Death Benefit is appropriate for:

   A. A beneficiary who is disabled, either physically or mentally

   B. A patient who is a homeowner aged 62 or older

   C. A patient who is terminally ill and has a life insurance policy he can sell to a third party

   D. A patient who is terminally ill and has a life insurance policy he can receive funds from during the terminal illness

21. Which answer best describes the impact of Medication Adherence?

    A. Nearly 50-75% of adults are medication non-adherent in one or more ways.

    B. 50% of hospital and skilled nursing admissions are due to medication nonadherence.

    C. Money is the most common cause of medication nonadherence.

    D. Approximately 1 in every 3 prescriptions are never filled.

Answer Key

1. Answer: D

Rationale: Screening is the first step in the case management process. During the screening step, patient information is reviewed to determine the appropriateness for case management.

Refer to: CCMC Glossary of Terms.

2. Answer: A

Rationale: The transitioning step of the case management process consists of activities such as assessing whether the client is ready for transfer to another level of care, facility, provider, or discharge to home (CCMC). Safety is the key concern with transitions of care.

Refer to: CCMC Glossary of Terms.

3. Answer: A

Rationale: Activities of Daily Living (ADLs) is an assessment tool that evaluates areas of essential function for self-care.

Refer to: CCMC Glossary of Terms.

4. Answer: C

Rationale: The Patient Health Questionnaire (PHQ-2) pre-screens patients for depression. Clients who pre-screen positive should be evaluated further with the Patient Health Questionnaire (PH-9)

Refer to: Subdomain–Physical Functioning and Behavioral Health Assessment.

5. Answer: C

Rationale: During a transition of care, a patient is at increased risk for adverse outcomes due to medication errors, failure to follow up on testing procedures, or not continuing prescribed medication treatments or therapies.

Refer to: Subdomain–Transitions of Care/Transitional Care.

6. Answer: D

Rationale: The interdisciplinary Care Team (ICT) is a group of healthcare professionals from various professional disciplines who work together to manage the physical, psychological and spiritual needs of the patient. Answers A, B, C, can be activities of a healthcare team.

Refer to: Subdomain–Interdisciplinary/Interprofessional Care Team.

7. Answer: B

Rationale: Hospice provides end of life care, which includes palliative care to patients with a terminal illness. Hospice care is a benefit covered under Medicare, Medicaid, and most private insurance companies.

Refer to: Subdomain–Hospice, Palliative, and End of Life Care.

8. Answer: C

Rationale: SSDI is an earned benefit that is funded by Social Security taxes paid by workers, employers, and the self-employed.

Refer to: Subdomain–Insurance Principles.

9. Answer: B

Rationale: Coordination of benefits prevents double payment for services when the subscriber has coverage from 2 or more sources. It determines which plan pays first.

Refer to: CCMC Glossary of Terms.

10. Answer: C

Rationale: An accountable care organization provides care through a network of providers. These providers coordinate patient care, minimize or eliminate duplicative services with a goal of improving clinical outcomes.

Refer to: Subdomain–Reimbursement and Payment Methodologies.

11. Answer: B

Rationale: A viatical settlement is when a person with a terminal or life-threatening illness and a life expectancy of less than 5 years, sells their insurance policy to a third party for cash.

Refer to: Subdomain—Financial Resources.

12. Answer: C

Rationale: Medicare Part D covers prescription drugs.

Refer to: Subdomain—Public Benefits Programs.

13. Answer: D

Rationale: Precertification is the process of obtaining and documenting advance approval from the health plan before delivering the needed medical services.

Refer to: CCMC Glossary of Terms.

14. Answer: C

Rationale: Workers' Compensation provides wage replacement and medical coverage for workers injured on the job and has no waiting period.

Refer to: Subdomain—Insurance Principles.

15. Answer: D

Rationale: Medicare covers an SNF stay if it follows within 30 days of a hospital stay of at least 3 days and is medically necessary. Answer C describes custodial care, Medicare only covers skilled services.

Refer to: Subdomain—Public Benefits Programs.

16. Answer: B

Rationale: In an EPO, patients are not reimbursed for out-of-network care.

Refer to: Subdomain—Healthcare Delivery Systems.

17. Answer: B

Rationale: They are asking for information on the patient's current status to determine medical necessity. This is characterized as a concurrent or continued stay review.

Refer to: Subdomain—Utilization Management Principles and Guidelines.

18. Answer: A

Rationale: A supplemental cost-sharing arrangement between the member and the insurer in which the member pays a specific charge for a specified service. Copayments may be flat or variable amounts per unit of service, and may be for such things as physician office visits, prescriptions, or hospital services. The payment is incurred at the time of service.

Refer to: CCMC Glossary of Terms.

19. Answer: A

Rationale: CCMC's website defines case management as "a collaborative process that assesses, plans, implements, coordinates, monitors, and evaluates the options and services required to meet the client's health and human service needs."

Refer to: CCMC website https://ccmcertification.org/about-ccmc/about-case-management/definition-and-philosophy-case-management

20. Answer: D

Rationale: An Accelerated Death Benefit rider is attached to an insurance policy and allows a patient to receive funds from the policy in the event of a terminal illness.

Refer to: Subdomain–Financial Resources.

21. Answer: A

Rationale: "A" is the most commonly cited statistic by the National Institute of Health; B is incorrect the statistic often cited is 20-25%; C is incorrect because the most common cause is thought to be lack of understanding/education about the importance of medication adherence; D, the CDC statistics indicate 1 in every 5 prescriptions are never filled.

Refer to: Subdomain–Adherence to Care Regimen.

Chapter Four:
Psychosocial Concepts
and Support Systems

Psychosocial Concepts and Support Systems comprise 25% of the exam with between 36 and 40 questions on this topic.

****

An effective case manager must understand everything that impacts the client and his ability to reach an optimal level of functioning. This includes, but is not limited to, support systems, psychosocial aspects, family dynamics, financial factors, culture, spirituality, and religion.

<<<< >>>>

Interpersonal Communication

Interpersonal communication is the process of exchanging ideas, thoughts, and feelings between individuals. Case managers must be skilled in communicating effectively with patients, family members, caregivers, providers, and team members. Interpersonal communication involves conveying information effectively but also requires active listening.

Active listening is a fundamental part of interpersonal communication. To listen effectively, avoid jumping to conclusions or making premature judgments. Active listening can be demonstrated by nodding the head, making eye contact, repeating what is said, or note-taking. Note-taking should be kept to a minimum, however, so as not to spend more time looking at the computer or notepad than at the person speaking. Ask open-ended questions whenever possible, as they provide more information, are considered less threatening, and develop trust.

There are four components to communication:

- Sender
- Message
- Receiver
- Context (e.g., values, health beliefs, cultural background, pain, etc.)

Barriers to effective communication include:

- Physical interference (e.g., background noise, a non-private setting)
- Psychological noise (e.g., pain, hunger, anger, anxiety)
- Barriers to processing information (e.g., information overload, educational deficit, cognitive deficit)
- Perceptual barriers (e.g., prejudices of the listener formed by his or her unique experiences, cultural background, and value system)
- Structural barriers (e.g., layers of bureaucracy or other difficulties in reaching the other person)

In addition to verbal and written communication, there is nonverbal communication. The case manager should be aware of the nonverbal communication she is both giving and receiving. For example, a client who avoids eye contact or looks away when answering questions may not be telling the truth. On the other hand, the case manager should be sure her own nonverbal communication is showing that she is actively listening to the client.

Build trust and rapport in communicating with clients by finding common ground, such as shared goals. Build trust over time by doing what you say you will do, when you say you will do it.

Communication with or within a group is more complex than communication with an individual due to group dynamics. Group dynamics are the way members of a group relate to each other and the way the group relates to those outside the group. Group dynamics include:

Roles – The roles and identities that develop within the group, such as leader, authority, participant, follower.

Norms – The acceptable standards of behavior within the group that are shared by group members.

Conformity – Adjusting one's behavior to align with the norms of the group.

Interview Tools and Techniques

The client interview is a purposeful conversation and a collaborative effort between the case manager and the client. The client interview is the primary manner for obtaining information about the client to create an effective care plan, so it is imperative that the information obtained be complete and accurate. Therefore, the case manager should have good interview skills. The following steps can be taken to facilitate a successful interview.

Preparation

The interview should be scheduled for a time when there are no anticipated interruptions for either the client or the case manager. When scheduling the interview, the case manager should let the client know approximately how much time to allow and what information will be required. For example: "Mr. Smith, we will take approximately 30 minutes and need a list of your current medications and physicians' names."

Prior to the interview, review available information from the client's chart, medical records, prior encounters, etc. However, the reviewed materials are not a substitute for the client interview.

Prevent interruptions or distractions by silencing cell phones, turning off the TV, closing the door, or any other appropriate action. If the interview is over the telephone, make sure the client is at a location where he will be comfortable talking about private health information. For example, if he is talking on a cell phone at the grocery store, arrange a time when the client will have privacy.

Introduction

The case manager should introduce herself, including her title and whom she is employed by. For example, an insurance case manager should reveal to the client that she works for the insurance company. The case manager should then explain her role and inform the patient about the purpose of the interview. The case manager should ask the patient how he would like to be addressed. It is also a good idea to inform the client why the case manager will be asking so many questions.

Establish Rapport

The case manager should create an environment that helps the client feel safe disclosing sensitive, personal information. He will feel more comfortable disclosing personal information, health history, problems, and concerns after positive rapport has been established. Do so by showing authentic interest in the client as a human being. Ask the client a question about his job, family, or interests.

Assessment

The case manager should start the interview by asking open-ended questions, giving the client the opportunity to tell his story. When the client is speaking, the case manager should actively listen. Guided questions can be used to get more specific information or to redirect the interview.

Summary

The case manager can close the interview by providing a summary of the information obtained and explaining the plan of care. The client and case manager should collaborate on goals.

Motivational Interview

The motivational interview is a collaborative, client-centered approach to interviewing that focuses on helping the client discover his motivation for change. This is done through identification, examination, and resolution of the ambivalence to change.

Principles of motivational interviewing include:
- Express empathy – See things as the client sees them.
- Support self-efficacy – Focus on the client's skills, strengths, and previous successes.
- Roll with resistance – Do not increase resistance by confronting the client when resistance occurs.
- Recognize discrepancy – Help the client see the discrepancy between where he is and where he wants to be, without judgment.

Motivational interviewing is designed to avoid confrontation. Instead, it focuses on collaboration and partnership between the client and the case manager which builds trust. The case manager and client do not have to agree on everything; they may respectfully maintain differing opinions. But rather than impose her ideas on the client, the case manager should draw ideas out of the client. Lasting change is more likely when the client discovers his own reasons, motivation, and skills to change. Ultimately it is up to the client to follow through with these changes.

The basic approach used in motivational interviewing can be remembered by the acronym OARS:

Open-ended questions – Help the client explore reasons and strategies for change.

Affirmations – Build rapport and help the client see himself in a positive way.

Reflections – Guide the client toward resolving ambivalence by focusing on the positive and negative aspects of changing or not changing.

Summaries – Show interest and understanding while calling attention to important points in the discussion.

Health Coaching and Counseling

Health coaching or counseling is secondary prevention, meaning that the client already suffers from a chronic disease. The goal of health coaching and counseling is to lessen the impact of the disease. Health coaching uses a coordinated and proactive approach to managing care for patients with chronic illness. Health coaches, or disease managers, take on a different role than traditional medical professionals. Rather than instruct patients on what they should do, the role of the health coach is to support, encourage, and empower patients to achieve their goals using evidence-based guidelines. Outcomes measured in health coaching include decreased emergency department visits and hospitalizations, adherence to guidelines, and/ or clinical measures such as maintaining blood pressure or Hemoglobin A1c level. Successful disease management results in a higher quality of life, lower healthcare costs, and clinical improvement for the client.

The Health Coaching Process

Establish a relationship – The case manager develops a positive rapport with the patient to foster trust.

Motivational interview – The case manager helps the patient discover which issues are most concerning. The case manager then engages the client to elicit "change talk" and to discover inner motivations to make the necessary changes. Change talk can be fostered by asking questions such as, "How does your condition interfere with things you like to do?" The goal is to increase the patient's awareness of the potential problems, consequences, and risks related to his unhealthy behavior, as well as to discover what motivates the patient.

Goal setting – The case manager assists the patient in setting goals and helps the patient discover options for achieving the goals. The case manager continues to monitor the patient's progress and focuses on successes toward the goals.

Client Engagement

Improved client engagement has been shown to result in better health outcomes, better quality of care, and improved patient safety. Client engagement has such an impact on health outcomes that the Affordable Care Act has identified it as an integral component of quality in Accountable Care Organizations (ACOs) and patient-centered medical homes. Client engagement involves the exchange of information between the client and provider, as well as the client taking an active role in care decisions.

Factors that can impact client engagement include:

- Motivation
- Attitudes
- Beliefs
- Knowledge
- Cognitive ability
- Education
- Health literacy
- Past experiences with the health system
- Degree of self-efficacy
- Trust between patient and provider

Client engagement involves the case manager building a therapeutic relationship with the client to gain his trust and maximize his involvement. The engaged client will be taking action, such as exercising regularly, taking medications as prescribed, or monitoring blood sugars.

When the client is engaged, the case manager is working with him, not merely talking to him. When a client is not engaged, it can seem as though the case manager is swimming against the current.

To engage the client, the case manager must understand what is important to him. What are his concerns, values, beliefs, and goals? It is easier to engage the client with this information in hand. The motivational interview can be used to obtain this knowledge.

**See more information on the motivational interview under Interview Tools and Techniques.

Client Activation and Readiness to Change

Client activation describes the knowledge, skills, ability, willingness, and confidence a person has that allows him to become actively engaged in managing his own health and healthcare. It is very specific to the client.

The terms client activation and client engagement are often confused or used interchangeably. Although they are similar, they are not the same. Client engagement builds on client activation with behaviors such as maintaining a healthy diet, exercising regularly, or obtaining preventive care.

Example: An activated client has the knowledge, skills, resources, and confidence to manage his diabetes. The engaged client monitors his blood sugars, maintains his diet, and exercises daily.

The Patient Activation Measure (PAM) was developed by Judith Hubbard of the University of Oregon to measure a client's activation level. Studies have shown that clients with higher PAM scores are better able to engage in their health, have better health outcomes, and lower healthcare costs.

Clients with lower PAM scores are more likely to feel overwhelmed with managing their health. They are also less likely to understand and have confidence in their role in their own healthcare. By understanding a client's level of activation, healthcare clinicians can create individualized care plans to increase activation and engagement.

The main reason patients do not change health behaviors is ambivalence because they:

- Are not ready
- Do not think they are able to change
- Do not have a plan
- Do not have support

Ways to increase activation include:
- Meeting clients where they are
- Personalizing care
- Educating
- Empowering
- Increasing confidence
- Breaking down actions into small, manageable steps

Behavioral Change Theories and Stages

For greater success in helping a client make positive changes, a case manager or health coach should determine where the client is in the 5 Stages of Change.

The 5 Stages of Change

1. Pre-contemplation
2. Contemplation
3. Preparation
4. Action
5. Maintenance

In the pre-contemplation stage, the individual does not intend to take action in the foreseeable future. He may not think about the change or he may be resistant to it. Pressuring the client at this stage is usually not effective. "I don't want to quit smoking."

In the contemplation stage, the individual considers a change in the next six months but has not committed to it. He may be open to information on the benefits of change and how to successfully do so. "I know I need to quit smoking, I just don't know how."

Preparation is when the individual actively plans to make a change within the next month. They may even have taken small steps toward change. "I got my nicotine patches today and have set my quit date."

Action is the stage when the individual has successfully made a change and has sustained it for less than six months. He will be seeking reinforcement and encouragement. "I have not had a cigarette in nine days."

When the change has been sustained for more than six months, maintenance has been achieved. Relapse can occur at any level, however.

Client Empowerment

The Case Management Society of America (CMSA) lists empowering the client as one of the roles and functions that case managers perform. A case manager empowers her client, as well as his family, caregivers, and members of the healthcare delivery team, by supporting and educating them so they can understand and access quality, efficient healthcare (CMSA, 2020).

By providing education on treatment options, community resources, insurance benefits, psychosocial concerns, and the role of the case manager, the client, caregiver, and healthcare delivery team can better problem-solve and explore options of care to achieve the desired outcomes. The empowered client is able to manage his care and practice self-advocacy, increasing adherence to the plan of care.

Client Self-care Management

Self-management in patients with chronic disease refers to their behaviors and the decisions they make that affect their health. Self-management support is the care and encouragement provided to people with chronic conditions (and their families) to help them manage their health on a daily basis, make informed decisions about care, engage in healthy behaviors, and direct their care. It involves collaboration between the client and case manager to foster ownership by the client.

Shared decision-making between the patient and provider requires the patient to be informed. Informed decision-making requires two-way communication between the patient and provider, wherein the patient's unique situation, beliefs, and priorities are discussed alongside the treatment options, so the patient can make the best treatment choice. It supports the ethical principle that patients have the right to decide what care is appropriate for them, including the right to accept or decline healthcare.

Case managers empower patients to be informed and active decision-makers in their healthcare. They encourage patients to practice self-advocacy by explaining treatment options and providing education on the disease or injury, community resources, and insurance coverage. The case manager never makes a decision for the client, but rather guides the client in decision-making.

Health Literacy

Health literacy is not simply the ability to read. Health literacy is the ability to obtain, communicate, process, and understand basic health information. It requires a complex set of reading, listening, analytical, and decision-making skills, as well as the ability to apply these skills to health situations. In addition to basic literacy skills, health literacy requires knowledge of health topics, such as how the body works and causes of disease. This is the foundation needed to understand treatment options and consent documents. Health literacy also requires numeracy skills such as calculating insulin dosage, measuring medication, understanding nutrition labels, and interpreting lab results. Even successful and well-educated people may have low health literacy.

The National Assessment of Adult Literacy measures the health literacy of adults living in the United States using four basic performance levels: Proficient, Intermediate, Basic, and Below Basic. Only 12% of the population was found to have a proficient health literacy level. This means that nearly 9 out of 10 adults in the United States are not proficient in understanding health-related information.

Knowing this can help case managers ask their clients better questions. Instead of asking, "Do you understand your discharge instructions?" It is more appropriate to ask specific questions about how they are taking their medications, when they are following up with their doctor, and which signs and symptoms to report. Case managers should also use common language, not medical terms, when speaking with patients.

Low health literacy has been linked to higher rates of hospitalization and emergency department usage, less frequent use of preventive services, and a greater likelihood of taking medicines incorrectly. People with limited health literacy are also more likely to have chronic conditions and are less able to manage them effectively. All of these outcomes are associated with higher healthcare costs.

Those at highest risk for low health literacy are:

- Older adults
- Racial and ethnic minorities
- Those having less than a high school degree or GED
- Individuals whose income is at or below poverty level
- Non-native speakers of English

Signs of low health literacy include deferring questions about their health history to a family member, stating that a family member handles their medications, frequent hospitalizations or emergency room visits, misuse of medications, and not being able to verbalize the plan of care.

The case manager can use single question assessments to assess health literacy, such as:

- How often do you have someone help you read hospital materials?

- How confident are you filling out medical forms by yourself?

- How often do you need to have someone help you when you read instructions, pamphlets, or other written material from your doctor or pharmacy?

There are also formal health literacy instruments. The most widely used are:

Rapid Estimate of Adult Literacy in Medicine (REALM) – Assesses the ability of adult patients to read common medical words and lay terms for illnesses and body parts. The examiner scores the patient on the number of words pronounced correctly, but no attempt is made to determine if the patient actually understands the meaning of the word. This assessment is only available in English.

The Newest Vital Sign – A tool that tests literacy skills for both numbers and words. It is designed to assess a patient's health literacy skills quickly and simply, taking only three minutes to administer. The patient is given a specially designed ice cream nutrition label to review and is asked a series of questions about it. Based on the number of correct answers, healthcare providers assess the patient's health literacy level. It is available in English and Spanish.

Test of Functional Health Literacy Assessment (TOFHLA) – A more complex assessment that takes 20 minutes or more to administer and consists of two parts, each with different types of questions.

The first part consists of 17 multiple choice questions that test a patient's ability to interpret numbers and documents. The second part assesses reading comprehension by asking patients to read three passages of text, in which a blank line replaces keywords. The patient chooses the word that makes the most sense from a word bank. A shorter version of the test is available and is known as the S-TOFHLA. It can be completed in about 12 minutes and contains four multiple choice questions and two reading passages. Both the TOFHLA and the S-TOFHLA are available in English and Spanish.

Wellness and Illness Prevention Programs, Concepts, and Strategies

Maintaining wellness and preventing disease can improve the length and quality of a patient's life. It can also be cost-effective. The case manager should assess the client for risk factors including diet and activity level, tobacco and alcohol use, as well as compliance with immunizations and screenings. Education should be provided when needed.

Many employers offer wellness programs through which participants are screened for risk factors and offered free education and support in areas where improvement is needed. Some of the more popular programs include smoking cessation, weight loss, and stress control.

Vaccines

Case managers may assess for updated vaccines, including the yearly flu vaccine, the pneumococcal vaccine, and the shingles vaccine. Patients with chronic conditions are particularly vulnerable to the flu and pneumonia.

Diet

Case managers should assess the patient's diet and access to proper nutrition. When a deficit is identified, the case manager can provide nutritional education and refer the patient to community resources.

Physical Activity

Engaging in regular physical activity is one of the most important factors in maintaining and improving health. Physical activity strengthens bones, increases muscle, reduces depression and stress, and helps maintain a healthy weight. Thirty minutes of moderate physical activity a day is recommended. Case managers can provide education and referrals to community resources to help clients find an activity that meets their needs.

Mammograms

The American Cancer Society recommends women age 40 and older have yearly mammograms.

Colorectal Cancer Screening

Men and women of average risk should begin screening for colorectal cancer at the age of 50.

Psychological and Neuropsychological Assessment

During the initial exam and on subsequent interactions with the client, case managers should assess:

- Temporary or permanent functional changes
- Physiological, psychological, or social problems
- Problems functioning in the community

If the need for further assessment is indicated, a referral for neuropsychological testing should be made. A medical evaluation should be performed prior to the psychological evaluation to rule out underlying medical conditions that can cause behavioral symptoms.

A neuropsychological evaluation should be performed on clients who have suffered a head injury to determine if there are any deficits. Neuropsychological testing is done by a neuropsychologist and includes a review of medical records, a personal interview, a review of psychiatric records, and psychological testing. Information is collected regarding the client's cognitive, behavioral, motor, linguistic, and executive functioning. If areas of deficits are found, a program can be created to address these areas.

Other Psychological, Neuropsychological, Functional, and Assessment Tools

Rancho Los Amigos Levels of Cognitive Functioning

The Rancho Los Amigos Scale of Cognitive Functioning is used to follow the recovery of the traumatic brain injury (TBI) patient. The scale is divided into eight stages, from coma to appropriate behavior and cognitive functioning. Those stages include:

I - Unresponsive to all stimuli

II - Generalized response to stimuli

III - Localized response to stimuli

IV - Confused/agitated

V - Confused/inappropriate, non-agitated behavior

VI - Confused/appropriate behavior

VII - Automatic/appropriate behavior

VIII - Purposeful/appropriate behavior

DSM-5

The Diagnostic and Statistical Manual of Mental Disorders (DSM-5) is the handbook used by healthcare professionals as the authoritative guide to the diagnosis of mental disorders. DSM-5 contains descriptions, symptoms, and other criteria for diagnosing mental disorders. It provides a common language for clinicians to communicate about their patients and establishes consistent and reliable diagnoses. DSM-5 is a manual for assessment and diagnosis of mental disorders but does not include information or guidelines for the treatment of any disorder.

Glasgow Coma Scale (GCS)

This assessment measures the level of coma in the acute phase of injury.

The Mini-Cog Test

A brief (approximately 3-minute) assessment instrument used to screen for cognitive impairment, Alzheimer's, and related dementia. The Mini-Cog involves two parts, a 3-item recall and a Clock Drawing Test (CDT), given in 3 steps.

Step 1: The person being tested is given the name of 3 common objects and is asked to repeat them back.

Step 2: They are asked to draw a clock showing a specified time. This serves as a recall distractor and a screening tool.

Step 3: The person is asked to name the 3 objects from Step 1.

The Mini-Mental Status Exam

An assessment of cognitive function consisting of 11 questions covering:
- Orientation
- Registration (immediate memory)
- Attention and calculation
- Recall
- Language and praxis

The test takes approximately 10 minutes to administer and can be used to help diagnose cognitive impairment following a head injury or the presence of dementia. It is also used to assess the severity and progression of the impairment. Scores of 25-30 are considered normal, and scores <24 are abnormal, with decreasing scores indicating increasing severity of impairment.

Hamilton-D

An assessment used by healthcare professionals to measure the level of depression of a client.

Minnesota Multiphasic Personality Inventory (MMPI)

The MMPI is a psychological test that assesses personality traits and psychopathology. It is most commonly used by mental health professionals to assess and diagnose mental illness. It can only be given and interpreted by a psychologist trained to do so.

Social Determinants of Health

The Centers for Disease Control and Prevention (CDC) lists 5 factors that contribute to a person's current state of health:
- Biology and genetics (e.g., sex and age)
- Individual behavior (e.g., alcohol use, injection drug use, unprotected sex, and smoking)
- Social environment (e.g., discrimination, income, and gender)
- Physical environment (e.g., where a person lives and crowding conditions)
- Health services (e.g., access to quality healthcare and having or not having health insurance)

Biology and genetics are fixed, but the remaining factors can be modified and together are known as the social determinants of health. The World Health Organization (WHO) defines social determinants of health as the conditions in which people are born, grow, live, work, and age. The social determinants of health are the factors that affect health outside of the hospital and doctor's office and include but are not limited to housing, social services, geographical location, and education.

Examples of social determinants include:

- Availability of resources to meet daily needs (e.g., safe housing and local food markets)
- Access to educational, economic, and job opportunities
- Access to healthcare services
- Availability of community-based resources in support of community living and opportunities for recreational and leisure-time activities
- Transportation options
- Social support
- Socioeconomic conditions (e.g., concentrated poverty and the stressful conditions that accompany it)
- Language/Literacy
- Access to mass media and emerging technologies (e.g., cell phones, the Internet, and social media)
- Exposure to toxic substances and other hazards
- Built environment, such as buildings, sidewalks, bike lanes, and roads

Let's take a closer look at how the social determinants of health may impact the clients we serve.

We know that poverty is a factor that can limit access to healthy foods, safe living conditions, and access to care, but it is important to remember, even where poverty is not a factor, social determinants of health impact the health of our clients. For example, a shortage of providers and specialists in the geographical area may result in long waits to access healthcare. Rural areas may not have the transportation options necessary for clients to access healthcare. Rural areas may also lack a public water source leaving residents using underground water sources that are potentially contaminated.

We will now take a deep dive into a few of the social determinants that impact the health of our clients.

Access to Healthcare

Many people face barriers that prevent or limit access to needed healthcare services, such as lack of health insurance, poor access to transportation, and limited healthcare resources.

Uninsured adults are less likely to receive preventive services or have a primary care physician. They often use emergency rooms for their healthcare needs. Insurance has been a major focus of our country's politics recently but having medical insurance alone does not guarantee the ability to afford healthcare. Out-of-pocket medical costs can still leave healthcare out of financial reach for many individuals causing them to delay or forgo needed care (such as doctor visits, dental care, and medications).

Lack of convenient and reliable transportation can also interfere with access to healthcare. Studies have shown that lack of transportation can lead to patients, especially those from vulnerable populations, delaying or skipping medication, rescheduling or missing appointments, and postponing care. Transportation barriers are also associated with a late-stage presentation of certain medical conditions (e.g., breast cancer).

Limited availability of healthcare resources is another barrier that may reduce access to health services and increase the risk of poor health outcomes. Physician shortages may mean that patients experience longer wait times and delayed care. Access issues arise for Medicaid patients when few physicians accept Medicaid due to their reduced reimbursement rates. And patients living in rural areas may not have easy access to hospitals, pharmacies, dialysis clinics, physicians, and other healthcare resources.

Speaking a language other than English at home can also impact access to healthcare. For example, a study found that Hispanic individuals who did not speak English at home were less likely to receive recommended preventive healthcare services for which they were eligible. Another study examined women of various racial and ethnic groups whose primary language was not English (they spoke Spanish, Cantonese, or Japanese) and found that they were less likely to be screened for breast or cervical cancer.

Another barrier to accessing healthcare is hours of availability. Most physicians' offices, testing centers, and clinics have limited office hours which may coincide with the work hours of the client. For a worker without sick leave benefits, missing work for a medical visit can result in lost wages or worse, losing their job.

Access to Foods that Support Healthy Eating Patterns

Studies show a relationship between the inability to access foods that support healthy eating patterns and negative health outcomes. For example, a study of 40,000 California residents looked into how access to healthy food choices impacts rates of obesity and diabetes. Residents of neighborhoods with fewer fresh produce sources and plentiful fast-food restaurants and convenience stores were at a higher risk of obesity and diabetes.

Low-income groups tend to rely on foods that are cheap and convenient to access but are low in nutrient density. Fresh fruits, vegetables, and other healthier items are often more expensive at convenience stores and small food markets than in larger chain supermarkets and grocery stores. A summary of recent research on this issue indicated that "in neighborhoods without supermarkets, residents likely face higher prices for many healthy foods because small stores typically charge more for items such as fresh produce." (Rose, 2010). Research also shows that price reductions of healthier food choices can contribute to increased purchasing of those choices.

Data from 2012—2013 show that the average distance from U.S. households to the nearest supermarket was 2.19 miles. Individuals without a vehicle or access to convenient public transportation, or who do not have food venues with healthy choices within walking distance, have limited access to foods that support healthy eating patterns. This can have a serious negative impact on those living in low-income and rural communities, especially older adults living in rural communities (Ver Ploeg, et al, 2015).

Environmental Conditions

Polluted air, contaminated water, and extreme heat are three of the many environmental conditions that can negatively impact health. The World Health Organization attributed 11% of U.S. mortality in 2012 (nearly 300,000 deaths) to environmental causes.

Poor water quality places the public's health at risk. Groundwater is the source of drinking water for nearly 1 out of 3 Americans, and in one study, 22% of public supply groundwater sources had at least one contaminant above recommended levels. In 2011–2012, 47% of waterborne illnesses were caused by untreated groundwater.

Housing Instability

Housing instability encompasses a number of challenges, such as having trouble paying rent, overcrowding, moving frequently, staying with relatives, homelessness, or spending the bulk of household income on housing. These experiences may negatively affect physical health and make it harder to access healthcare.

Households are considered to be cost-burdened if they spend more than 30% of their income on housing and severely cost-burdened if they spend more than 50% of their income on housing. Cost-burdened households have little left over each month to spend on other necessities such as food, clothing, utilities, and healthcare. People with the lowest incomes may be forced to rent substandard housing that exposes them to health and safety risks such as vermin, mold, water leaks, and inadequate heating or cooling systems. They may also be forced to move in with others, potentially resulting in overcrowding. Overcrowding may affect mental health, stress levels, relationships, and sleep, and it may increase the risk of infectious disease.

Moving three or more times in a year, often called "multiple moves," has been associated with negative health outcomes in children. Children who move frequently are more likely to have chronic conditions and poor physical health.

Impact for case managers

Patients affected by the social determinants of health are often those that need the case manager the most, as they can benefit considerably from case management services. They are the clients you will see in the ED over and over. They are the clients who will be labeled as "non-compliant" because they cannot follow the treatment plan. They are the clients who result in less than optimal outcomes for the case manager and healthcare organization if the social determinant of health is not addressed. By knowing and understanding how the social determinants of health impact clients and the resources available to them, the case manager is able to come up with creative resource solutions.

Psychosocial Aspects of Chronic Illness and Disability

How an individual is affected by chronic illness and disability may be influenced by numerous factors, including:

- Age
- Gender
- Race
- Culture
- Extent of functional limitation
- Prognosis
- Coping styles
- Past experiences
- Sense of self-efficacy

- Social support
- Family support
- Socioeconomic status

The effects of chronic illness and disability are individual and involve:

- Social and family relationships
- Economic well-being
- Activities of daily living
- Social activities
- Work activities
- Grief
- Distortion of body image

A disability is considered chronic when the impaired function will never be completely eliminated. The case manager should assess not only the physical effects of chronic illness or disability but also the psychosocial effects on both the patient and his family and caregivers. A chronic disability changes the client's self-perception and role. Case managers must understand the patient's role in the family (such as breadwinner or caregiver) and how that role is affected by the illness or disability. This will help the case manager understand the impact of the illness or disability. The case manager can then design a plan of care to educate, support, and counsel the patient to manage symptoms, carry out treatments, and make lifestyle and behavior changes.

Self-efficacy

Self-efficacy is one's belief in their own ability to succeed, and it plays a major role in the client's outcome. The more self-efficacy a client possesses, the more likely he will persevere when obstacles arise. For a behavioral change to take hold, the client must know what to do, believe it is beneficial, and believe it is attainable.

Factors that influence self-efficacy include the client's physiological and psychological state, mastery of experiences, vicarious experiences, and social persuasion. With each experience the client masters, he finds evidence that he has the ability to succeed. Witnessing others in similar situations overcome their obstacles is further proof that perseverance can lead to success. Continuous positive persuasion strengthens personal beliefs regarding success.

The case manager can foster and encourage self-efficacy in the client in many ways. She can provide affirmation, motivation, and encouragement. She can facilitate goal setting that will promote mastery by helping the client create small, attainable goals. Many disabled individuals have made major contributions to society. The case manager can tell these individuals' stories to remind the client what is possible. She can also assist the client reach optimal physical and psychological function by making referrals as needed.

Client Support System Dynamics

When a person becomes ill or injured there are numerous implications; financially, emotionally, physically, and socially. The client's family is usually his source of support, and when necessary, his caregiver. Families provide the majority of long-term care for patients. To best serve the patient, case managers need to provide support and advocacy for the family as well as the patient.

To best assess the situation, the case manager needs to understand the client's role in the family. Was he the breadwinner? Was he the caregiver to another family member? How does his illness affect this role? No matter the client's role in the family, the illness or injury will disrupt the family norms. An extended or severe illness will require modifications of family responsibilities.

Case managers also need to understand the family's dynamics. Many families have issues that can affect their ability to adapt to a crisis situation such as an illness or injury. Are family members dealing with alcoholism, mental illness, depression, abuse, or their own health issues? Is this an intact family or a divorced family with stepparents, stepchildren, and/or step siblings? Issues that existed before will be intensified during times of stress.

An adaptive family is able to adjust to crisis; this is important to help the patient reach his goals. An adaptive family possesses the ability to:

- Be flexible
- Problem solve
- Communicate effectively
- Seek and accept help

A maladaptive family is unable to meet the changing needs of the family. Maladaptive families:

- Overindulge the patient
- Foster patient dependency
- Abandon other family members
- Abandon the patient
- Deny the patient's condition
- Rely on a single person to provide all assistance to the patient
- Fail to seek assistance or ask for help

The case manager's ability to understand the family dynamics will assist her in providing interventions and resources as needed. She can make a referral to family counseling or support groups. She can also encourage the family to maintain as much of their normal routine as possible, to take care of themselves, and to ask for help.

Assessing for caregiver support and family coping is an ongoing process. Everyone may come together initially and set aside family issues, but maladaptive family dynamics may surface later. The primary caregiver may become burned out as initial support may diminish over time.

Supportive Care Programs

Initial and ongoing assessments should be conducted to identify additional support needs. If needs are identified, the case manager can refer the patient to one of the many local and national disease-based programs to provide education, financial resources, and peer support. The American Cancer Society, for example, offers patients assistance with lodging when traveling for care away from home, local transportation to and from treatments and appointments, and online support groups, along with many other resources.

Support programs are also available for caregivers. Many communities have local support groups, and national organizations, such as the Alzheimer's Foundation of America, offer support services and strategies for caregivers.

For patients with deeply held spiritual beliefs (identified during the spiritual assessment upon enrollment in case management), pastoral counseling may be an integral part of their treatment.

Bereavement counseling can aid in the loss of a loved one, as well as other losses brought on by illness or tragedy. Local hospice agencies are a good resource for bereavement counseling and will provide this service to anyone, not just their clients.

Resources for the Uninsured or Underinsured Including Community Resources

Like the uninsured, the underinsured may have difficulty obtaining healthcare. For example, if an individual has medical insurance but no prescription coverage, he can see the doctor and get a diagnosis and prescription to treat the problem, but he may not be able to afford to fill the prescription. A client suffering a stroke may exhaust a 30-visit limit for outpatient rehabilitation long before reaching his maximum potential.

Even with the best insurance coverage, some services are not covered, such as home modifications, caregivers, healthy meals, and transportation to doctor appointments. Case managers often need to remove barriers to care by referring clients to available resources beyond their health benefit, such as community resources. Community resources are also available for caregivers, providing support and respite.

Fraternal and religious organizations often offer a variety of resources ranging from building wheelchair ramps to food pantries. The Area Agency on Aging assists clients 60 or older and those with disabilities to live in their homes and communities for as long as possible by providing services in the five categories below.

Information and access services:
- Health insurance counseling
- Information and referral assistance
- Transportation
- Caregiver support
- Retirement planning education

Community-based services:
- Employment services
- Adult day care
- Senior centers
- Group meals

In-home services:
- Meals on wheels
- Homemakers
- Telephone reassurances
- Energy assistance and weatherization

- Home health services
- Respite care
- Personal care services

Housing:

- Senior housing
- Alternative community-based living facilities

Elder rights:

- Legal assistance
- Elder abuse prevention programs
- Ombudsman services

Meal delivery can help an elderly person maintain independence and continue living at home. The Meals On Wheels Association of America is a national network of more than 5,000 Senior Nutrition Programs that operate in all 50 states delivering nutritious meals to seniors.

People with limited income may have to choose between food and their medications. Nearly all communities have local food banks to provide nutritious food for needy members of the community. In addition, many drugstores and grocery store chains have programs that allow patients to refill their generic medications for free or a nominal fee. Some pharmaceutical companies offer pharmacy assistance programs, through which some of their medications can be obtained by uninsured or low-income individuals at a discount or no cost. Many states also have pharmacy assistance programs for seniors and other qualifying individuals.

Lack of transportation can impact access to healthy food, the ability to refill prescriptions, and access to healthcare. The types of transportation available will vary widely based on location. Many metropolitan areas have numerous transportation options such as bus, taxi, Uber/Lyft (rideshare), rail, and/or subway. Rural and suburban areas can be more challenging.

Some local communities, nonprofits, and faith-based organizations offer transportation for the elderly and disabled. These may be paid drivers or volunteers.

Other community resources include:
- Disease organizations (e.g., American Cancer Society, MS Society, National Kidney Fund, Alzheimer's Association)
- Charity organizations (e.g., United Way)
- Service organizations (e.g., Rotary, Elks, Lions Club)
- Make-A-Wish
- American Association of Retired Persons (AARP)
- Public Health Departments

In addition to the resources above, government programs, such as the Katie Beckett Waiver and the Children's Health Insurance Program (CHIP), may help.

The Katie Beckett Waiver enables severely disabled children and adults to be cared for at home and be eligible for Medicaid based on the affected individual's income and assets alone. Without the waiver, the income of legally liable relatives is counted when the individual is cared for at home.

The Children's Health Insurance Program (CHIP) provides health coverage to children in families with incomes too high to qualify for Medicaid, but who do not have, and can't afford, private health insurance coverage. Other programs are available and vary from state to state.

Behavioral Health Concepts And Symptoms

Dual Diagnosis/Co-occurring Disorders

Dual diagnosis, or co-occurring disorder, describes patients with coexisting mental illness and substance abuse disorders. The mental illness must meet the criteria for diagnosis by the Diagnostic and Statistical Manual of Mental Disorders (DSM-5, 2013). Dual diagnoses are not uncommon, with about half of those with a severe mental illness and one-third of those with mental illness also struggling with substance abuse. The prognosis for patients with mental illness who abuse drugs and/or alcohol is worse than for patients who do not.

Psychiatric treatment is more successful with patients who are not actively abusing these substances. For this reason, the first step is often for the patient to stop using—or, if the patient is addicted, to detox the patient. Additional treatment may include individual counseling, support groups, and medications to help the patient develop coping skills, build self-confidence, and manage the symptoms of mental illness.

Patients with dual diagnoses are often a challenge for case managers. They are less likely to follow through with their treatment plan by missing appointments and failing to take medications. The case manager will find greater success if she can help the patient find the motivation to comply with the treatment plan.

Substance Use, Abuse, and Addiction

Substance use includes alcohol, over the counter drugs, prescription drugs, and illegal drugs. Substance use does not equal substance abuse.

The American Psychiatric Association's Diagnostic and Statistical Manual of Mental Disorders, 5th Edition (DSM-5) defines substance abuse as a maladaptive pattern of substance use leading to clinically significant impairment or distress, as manifested by one (or more) of the following, occurring within a 12-month period:

- Recurrent substance use resulting in a failure to fulfill major role obligations at work, school, or home (e.g., repeated absences or poor work performance related to substance use; suspensions or expulsions from school; neglect of children or household)
- Recurrent substance use in situations in which it is physically hazardous (e.g., driving an automobile when impaired by substance use)

- Recurrent substance-related legal problems (e.g., arrests for substance-related disorderly conduct)
- Continued substance use despite having persistent or recurrent social or interpersonal problems caused or exacerbated by the effects of the substance (e.g., arguments with spouse about consequences of intoxication; physical fights)

The case manager must assess for substance abuse or addiction since it may complicate the diagnosis and/or treatment of medical conditions. Most patients will not readily admit that they have an addiction problem. The CAGE tool is available for screening substance abuse. It consists of four questions:

1. "Have you ever felt you should **C**ut down on drinking/drug use?"

2. "Have people **A**nnoyed you by criticizing your drinking/drug use?"

3. "Have you ever felt **G**uilty about your drinking/drug use?"

4. "Have you ever taken a drink/used drugs in the morning to steady your nerves or get rid of a hangover (**E**ye opener)?"

Answering yes to two of the questions provides strong indication for substance abuse. Answering yes to three of the questions confirms the likelihood of substance abuse or dependency.

Withdrawal from alcohol and drugs can cause anxiety, tachycardia, tremors, grand mal seizures, insomnia, nausea and/or vomiting, and hallucinations. Detoxification treats these physical effects.

The case manager's role is to support the treatment plan, provide encouragement to the patient and his family/caregivers, and refer to AA or similar organizations.

Levels of care for addiction are based on the program's structure, including the setting, intensity, and frequency of services.

Level I: Outpatient Treatment

Less than 9 hours per week of directed treatment and recovery services.

Level II: Intensive/Partial Hospitalization Treatment

Regularly scheduled sessions for a minimum of 9 hours per week in a structured program, with the opportunity for the client to interact in his own environment.

Level III: Medically Monitored Intensive Inpatient

Inpatient treatment with 24-hour observation, monitoring, and treatment by a multidisciplinary staff.

Level IV: Medically Managed Intensive Inpatient

Medical and nursing services along with the full resources of a hospital, available on a 24-hour basis.

Community-based programs such as Alcoholics Anonymous and Narcotics Anonymous have been found to be the most successful in treating substance abuse. Inpatient hospitalization for substance abuse is not usually the preferred method of treatment.

Crisis Intervention Strategies

A crisis can refer to any situation in which the client perceives the inability to effectively problem-solve and/or cope. A situation that is a crisis to one individual may not be a crisis to another. Not all crises involve danger, but if the patient is in danger, the first priority is his safety. Get professional help, even if the patient resists. Never leave him alone. If he is admitted to an inpatient facility, he will require 1:1 observation.

If at any time the patient is thought to be at risk for suicide, the case manager should ask directly if he has a plan to commit suicide. If there is any doubt about the patient's safety, he should be admitted. If safety is not an issue, help him develop good support systems or refer him to a support group, counselor, therapist, or psychiatrist as appropriate. Remove items such as weapons or large quantities of medications from the patient's access. Complete frequent follow-up assessments to evaluate the effectiveness of the interventions.

Suicide risk factors include:
- History of prior suicide attempt
- Family history of suicide
- Living alone
- Recently divorced or widowed
- History of mental illness
- Chronic illness
- History of substance abuse
- Unemployed
- Recent loss
- Hopelessness or helplessness
- Risk-taking behavior
- Giving away prized possessions
- Lack of interest in future plans

After safety is established, listen to the client to assess his state of need. Always allow him to tell his story and express his full emotions without the fear of being judged. Assist the client to assess available resources and strategies that have worked for him in the past. Collaborate on finding alternative coping mechanisms and setting goals, while focusing on the client's strengths.

Conflict Resolution Strategies

When faced with a conflict, it is important for all parties to focus on the goal, rather than the person or persons they are in conflict with. It is also important to keep communication open and to avoid bringing emotion and/or reactivity into the process. If the case manager believes emotion or reaction are taking over, it is best to call for a "cooling off period" where both parties can take a break, resuming when the focus can be placed back on the goal.

The following five conflict resolution strategies are listed from most to least desirable for most situations. Remember that the situation will dictate the best conflict resolution strategy to utilize.

1. Collaboration – This strategy meets the needs of all parties involved.

2. Negotiation – Finding a solution that gives everyone a partial win, with everyone giving something up. This strategy is most useful when there is a standstill in negotiations and the parties are approaching a deadline.

3. Accommodation – This meets the needs of the other party at the expense of one's own needs.

4. Competitive – This style takes a firm stand. It is useful in emergency situations when decisions need to be made fast. It can also be utilized when someone is trying to take advantage of a situation. When used inappropriately, however, this strategy can leave the other party feeling resentful, bullied, or unsatisfied.

5. Avoidance – This style avoids the conflict by allowing the default action.

Multicultural, Spiritual, and Religious Factors

Culture consists of languages, beliefs, values, traditions, and customs. The case manager is to practice cultural competence with awareness and respect for diversity. She should be aware of, and responsive to, cultural and demographic diversity of the population. Case managers are to take part in ongoing cultural competency training to enhance their work with multicultural populations.

A cultural assessment, including an assessment of the client's linguistic needs, should be included in the case manager's initial client assessment. While it is necessary for a case manager to understand general cultural norms as they relate to healthcare, it is more important that she understands that each patient is an individual with his own individual, family, and cultural beliefs. Sometimes these cultural beliefs conflict with the treatment plan. When this happens the case manager should attempt to adjust the treatment plan to work within the cultural limits. If this is not possible, the case manager must educate the client on the possible effects of not complying with the treatment plan. This should be done respectfully without coercing the client. Ultimately, it is the client who chooses to follow the treatment plan.

At times, the client's cultural beliefs may be very different from the case manager's. This can influence how a case manager views her clients. The case manager must respect the client's beliefs, even though she may not agree with them. It can be helpful to acknowledge cultural differences with the client, and reassure the client that the case manager's job is to educate him and support his decisions.

Case managers should assess the client's linguistic needs and identify resources to enhance proper communication. This may include the use of interpreters and material in different languages and formats. When using an interpreter it is best to use a professional interpreter—not a family member—whenever possible.

Spirituality is a broad concept with many perspectives. In general, it includes a sense of connection to something bigger than us, and it typically involves a search for meaning in life. For some people, spirituality is synonymous with religion, but a person does not have to have a religious belief to be spiritual.

It is important to have an understanding of clients' spiritual and religious views, as the views often impact choices they make in regard to healthcare.

For example, if a patient believes that he has no control over his destiny, he may feel that lifestyle changes or medical intervention will not change the inevitable, and therefore decline treatment or lifestyle changes. On the other hand, if the patient believes that life is precious and all means should be exhausted in prolonging it, he may be unwilling to accept the withdrawal of life-sustaining treatment, even when death is inevitable. It is also important to understand that some religious beliefs can affect healthcare choices; for example, Jehovah's Witnesses do not accept blood transfusions and some Pentecostal Christians will refuse medical treatment due to their strong belief in miraculous healing.

Assessing a patient's spiritual needs is an important part of the initial assessment with the client. With this information the case manager can refer the patient to resources for spiritual counseling. During times of illness, patients often rely on their spiritual beliefs to cope. Spiritual practices tend to improve coping skills, provide optimism and hope, promote healthy behavior, decrease feelings of depression and anxiety, and encourage a sense of relaxation. By relieving stressful feelings and promoting healing ones, spirituality can positively influence immune, cardiovascular, hormonal, and nervous systems. Studies have shown that terminally ill patients with a higher spiritual well-being were less likely to have depression and thoughts of suicide.

Case managers should avoid judging a patient's healthcare decision based on spiritual beliefs. When possible the case manager can offer alternatives that are within the patient's beliefs.

Gender Health

The following definitions come from the Oxford Dictionary (http://english. oxforddictionaries.com/):

> Gender Identity: a person's perception of having a particular gender, which may or may not correspond with their birth sex.

Gender Expression: the way in which a person expresses their gender identity, typically through their appearance, dress, and behavior.

Sexual Orientation: a person's sexual identity in relation to the gender to which they are attracted; the fact of being heterosexual, homosexual, or bisexual.

For ease of reading, we use "transgender." However, the information can be applied to all gender non-conforming people.

There has been very little research on transgender people and their health needs. However, from what has been studied, we do know that they experience a great deal of misunderstanding, rejection, and discrimination, all of which can lead to poor health outcomes.

Barriers to healthcare include:

- Name on insurance card and medical records not matching identified name
- Denial of routine preventive care for body parts not consistent with gender on record
- Denial of medically necessary treatment if the sex on file with insurance does not match anatomy
- Lack of healthcare providers trained in transgender medical and behavioral healthcare
- Fear of, or actual discrimination or humiliation
- Lack of health insurance

Ideally, healthcare organizations should have a system that allows patients to input their preferred name, gender, and pronouns on registration forms and other relevant documents. This allows all staff to see the patients' preferences, and to use them consistently. Creating such a system is helpful for non-transgender patients as well, since some patients might prefer to use nicknames or middle names, etc.

If your organization does not collect this information, you can ask "How would you like to be addressed?" or "What name do you go by?" Once a patient has given a preferred name, it is very important for staff to use this name in all interactions.

Abuse and Neglect

There are numerous types of abuse and neglect, including physical, emotional/psychological, sexual, financial, and medical neglect. The elderly are at increased risk for abuse, with those over age 80 at the highest risk. The perpetrators of abuse and neglect are most often family members, with the majority of them being spouses and adult children. As case managers are often in contact with the caregivers, they should be aware of the risk factors of abusers. These risk factors include mental illness, alcohol and drug abuse, history of abuse, inability to cope with stress, depression, lack of support from other potential caregivers, and caregiver reluctance.

If the case manager identifies that the patient is at increased risk, she can try interventions that may reduce the threat of abuse.

- Ensure the caregiver receives proper training and education on his or her responsibilities
- Help the caregiver develop a support system and identify support groups and respite care
- Inquire about situations that frustrate or anger the caregiver and help him or her identify appropriate responses
- If necessary, assist with the arrangement for paid caregivers or placement of the patient in the appropriate long-term care setting

Nurses are mandated reporters of abuse or neglect. If abuse or neglect is suspected, they must notify Adult Protective Services. Depending on the case, the police may also be notified. The case manager should carefully document all communication and findings objectively.

General Signs and Symptoms of Abuse and Neglect:

- Changes in personality or behavior
- Sudden change in physical or financial status
- Tension or arguments between caregiver and client
- Failure to take medications (or not refilling in appropriate time frame)
- Caregiver's refusal to allow elder to be seen alone

Types of Abuse and Neglect

Neglect – The failure or inability to provide for basic needs. This can be intentional or unintentional.

Emotional/Psychological Abuse – The infliction of anguish, pain, or distress through verbal or nonverbal acts, such as gestures or writing, resulting in trauma. This also includes threats of harm used to intimidate a person into complying or cooperating.

Examples of emotional and psychological abuse and neglect include:

- Verbal assaults
- Insults
- Threats
- Intimidation
- Humiliation or embarrassment
- Harassment
- Disregarding needs
- Damaging or destroying property
- Isolation
- Ridicule
- Coercion
- Mental cruelty

- Inappropriate sexual comments
- Controlling behavior (such as prohibiting or limiting access to transportation, telephone, money, or other resources)

Physical Abuse – The use of physical force, such as hitting, beating, pushing, shaking, slapping, kicking, burning, and pinching, that results in physical pain, bodily injury, or impairment. Also included in physical abuse is force-feeding and the use of drugs and physical restraints.

Signs of physical abuse and neglect include:

- Dehydration
- Poor hygiene and/or grooming
- Weight loss
- Unexplained bruises, burns, scars, broken bones, or sprains
- Restraint marks
- Skin breakdown
- Vaginal or rectal pain
- Abrasions, bleeding, or bruising in the genital area
- Lab results showing overdose of medication

Financial Abuse and Neglect – Failing to use the patient's income or assets for the benefit, support, and maintenance of the patient. The illegal, unauthorized, or improper use of the resources of the patient.

Examples of financial abuse and neglect include:

- Forgery
- Theft
- Coercion
- Deception
- Fraud

BONUS

For inspiration, support, and encouragement to help you pass the CCM exam, as well as to grow in the profession, we have a Facebook group with over 14,000 case managers that I would like to personally invite you to join. Search for *Case Managers Community* on Facebook, or find the link on the website associated with this book,

CCMcertificationMadeEasy.com

References

American Psychiatric Association, DSM-5 Task Force. (2013). *Diagnostic and statistical manual of mental disorders: DSM-5™* (5th ed.). American Psychiatric Publishing, Inc. https://doi.org/10.1176/appi.books.9780890425596

Case Management Society of America. (2016). *Standards of practice for case management.* http://solutions.cmsa.org/acton/media/10442/standards-of-practice-for-case-management

Centers for Disease Control and Prevention. (n.d.). https://www.cdc.gov/

Commission for Case Management Certification. (2017). *Glossary of terms.* https://ccmcertification.org/get-certified/exam-study-materials/ccmc-glossary

Oxford University Press. (n.d.). *Lexico.* Retrieved June 11, 2020, from http://english.oxforddictionaries.com/

Rose, D. (2010) Access to healthy food: A key focus for research on domestic food insecurity. The Journal of Nutrition. 2010 Jun;140(6):1167–69. https://doi.org/10.3945/jn.109.113183

Ver Ploeg, M., Mancino, L., Todd, J.E., Clay, D.M., & Scharadin, B. (2015). Where do Americans usually shop for food and how do they travel to get there? Initial findings from the national household food acquisition and purchase survey. United States Department of Agriculture Economic Research Service; 2015 Mar. 27 p. EIB-138.

World Health Organization. (2016, March). *An estimated 12.6 million deaths each year are attributable to unhealthy environments.* https://www.who.int/news-room/detail/15-03-2016-an-estimated-12-6-million-deaths-each-year-are-attributable-to-unhealthy-environments

<<<< >>>>

Test Your Knowledge On Psychosocial Concepts and Support Systems

1. Barriers to effective communication include all but which of the following:

   A. Physical interference from the environment

   B. Cognitive deficits

   C. Open-ended questions

   D. Cultural factors

2. What is the best description of Client Engagement?

   A. The engaged client listens but does not act.

   B. The engaged client accepts advice and guidance without question or discussion with the healthcare team.

   C. An engaged client shares information with the healthcare team and takes an active role in care decisions.

   D. An engaged client is unwilling to discuss cultural requirements impacting healthcare outcomes.

3. The case manager supports Client Empowerment through all the following actions except:

   A. Providing client-specific education and resources

   B. Encouraging shared decision making

   C. Collaborating with the client and the healthcare team

   D. Creating detailed lists for the client to follow

4. The Motivational Interviewing principle of expressing empathy is best explained by which of the following:

   A. Help the client see the discrepancy between where he is and where he wants to be

B. Focus on the client's skills, strengths, and previous successes

C. Seeing things as the client sees them through reflective listening

D. Using a collaborative, client-centered approach to interviewing focuses on helping the client discover his motivation for change

5. Health literacy is more than the ability to read. All of the following are aspects of health literacy except:

A. Basic literacy skills

B. Basic English competency

C. Basic knowledge of how the body works

D. Basic math skills

6. Shared decision making is best exemplified by which scenarios below?

A. Information about self-care measures are provided to a client caregiver

B. Treatment options are decided between the case manager and the provider

C. Clients choose what treatment options they prefer after education from the case manager and provider

D. Decisions made by clients must be geared toward the most therapeutic medical approach.

7. After suffering this type of injury/incident, a Neuropsychological evaluation is often required:

A. Myocardial Infarction

B. Traumatic Brain Injury

C. Amputation

D. Psychotic episode

8. By providing which of the following to the client is the case manager helping to foster self-efficacy?

    A. Resources for financial support

    B. Past experiences

    C. Social support

    D. Affirmation

9. Which factor below is the best indication a family is adapting to changing dynamics?

    A. Siblings are sent to live with other family members

    B. Parents are unable to coordinate caregiver help

    C. Stress levels are managed within the family unit

    D. Communication lines are closed to certain family members

10. Which tool can case managers use to assess for substance abuse or addiction?

    A. CAGE Tool

    B. Glasgow Coma Scale

    C. The Mini-Mental Exam

    D. Hamilton D

11. Mr. Brown lives with his adult daughter and her husband. He tells the case manager that he has not taken one of his blood pressure meds in a week because he ran out and cannot afford to refill it. He goes on to state his checkbook is missing several checks and his account is overdrawn. Mr. Brown is most likely:

    A. Suffering from dementia

    B. The victim of financial abuse

C. The victim of elder abuse

D. Making excuses for not taking his medications

12. Health coaching's purpose is to:

A. Educate clients about their disease

B. Instruct clients on disease prevention

C. Support, encourage and empower clients to reach their goals

D. Decrease ED visits and hospital admissions

13. Clients with mental illness such as depression and bipolar disease are at high risk for:

A. Dual diagnosis

B. Hospitalization

C. Obesity

D. Abuse and neglect

14. Mr. Williams is a 72-year-old male client with a low-income. He has been losing weight since his wife's death 6 months ago. He states he does not like to cook and has been living off of junk food since her death. The best resource for Mr. Williams is:

A. A meal delivery service

B. A housekeeper/cook

C. A cooking class

D. An assisted living facility

15. The first thing for the case manager to do when a client is not compliant with the plan of care is to:

A. Close the member to case management

B. Discuss barriers to compliance with the member

C. Notify the client's physician

D. Request a mental evaluation

16. Mary is a 37-year-old mother of two who is paralyzed from the waist down after a motor vehicle accident. She tells her case manager, "I can never be a good mom from this wheelchair." The case manager should:

A. Ignore the comment

B. Encourage the patient to explore her feelings regarding this

C. Tell the client she is lucky to be alive and should be thankful

D. Report her to social services

17. When the case manager becomes aware of a client's cultural or religious beliefs that conflict with the treatment plan, the case manager should:

A. Close the client to case management, the case manager will not be able to benefit the client

B. Try to convince the client to disregard their beliefs, science has proven them wrong

C. Attempt to adjust the treatment plan to work within the cultural/religious limits

D. Educate the client on the scientific evidence for the treatment plan

18. The case manager is working with a client in a weight loss program. The client makes the statement, "I have thrown out all of the unhealthy food in the house. I also started collecting healthy recipes and am ready to start my new way of eating on Monday." The case manager knows the client is in which stage of change?

A. Pre-Contemplation

B. Action

C. Preparation

D. Contemplation

Answer Key

1. Answer: C

   Rationale: Open-ended questions encourage effective communication; environmental interference, cognitive deficits, and cultural factors are all potential barriers to effective communication.

   Refer to: Subdomain–Interpersonal Communication.

2. Answer: C

   Rationale: An engaged client shares information with the healthcare team and takes an active role in decisions about their care. The other scenarios are signs of a disengaged client and present an opportunity for the case manager to find out why.

   Refer to: Subdomain–Client Engagement.

3. Answer: D

   Rationale: Creating detailed lists for the client to follow does not support empowerment because it doesn't foster self-advocacy or help him manage his own care. Providing client-specific education and resources, encouraging shared decision making, and collaborating with the client and healthcare team, empower the client, and increases adherence to the care plan.

   Refer to: Subdomain–Client Empowerment.

4. Answer: C

   Rationale: Empathy is seeing things as the client sees them. Expressing empathy is one of the four principles of Motivational Interviewing.

   Refer to: Subdomain–Interview Tools and Techniques.

5. Answer: B

   Rationale: While non-native English speakers are at a higher risk for low health literacy rates, a translator should be used and it doesn't determine health literacy alone. All other answers are required for being Health Literate.

Refer to: Subdomain–Health Literacy.

6. Answer: C

Rationale: "C" exemplifies shared decision making; A and B exclude the client in decision making; D does not allow the client to decline or modify treatment options.

Refer to: Subdomain–Client Self-care Management.

7. Answer: B

Rationale: A neuropsychological evaluation should be performed on clients who have suffered a head injury to determine if there are any deficits.

Refer to: Subdomain–Psychological and Neuropsychological Assessments.

8. Answer: D

Rationale: The case manager can foster and encourage self-efficacy in the client in many ways. She can provide affirmation, motivation, and encouragement.; A & C may be provided by the case manager but do not foster self-efficacy. B is incorrect because past experiences cannot be altered

Refer to: Subdomain–Psychosocial Aspects of Chronic Illness and Disability.

9. Answer: C

Rationale: Stress levels being managed indicate the family is adapting to changing dynamics. The other options are signs of a maladaptive family. The case manager's ability to understand the family dynamics will assist her in providing interventions and resources as needed.

Refer to: Subdomain–Client Support System Dynamics.

10. Answer: A

Rationale: The CAGE Tool is what is used for screening for substance abuse.

Refer to: Subdomain–Behavioral Health Concepts and Symptoms.

11. Answer: B

Rationale: The elderly are at increased risk of abuse. The perpetrators of abuse are most often family members. Financial abuse includes the unauthorized use of resources.

Refer to: Subdomain–Abuse and Neglect.

12. Answer: C

Rationale: Health coaching uses a coordinated and proactive approach to manage care for patients with chronic illness. Rather than instructing patients on what they should do, health coaches assist patients to achieve their healthcare goals. The role of the health coach is to support, encourage, and empower patients to achieve their goals.

Refer to: Subdomain–Health Coaching and Counseling.

13. Answer: A

Rationale: Dual diagnosis describes patients with coexisting mental illness and substance abuse disorders. One-third of those with mental illness also struggle with substance abuse.

Refer to: Subdomain–Behavioral Health Concepts and Symptoms.

14. Answer: A

Rationale: Home delivery services, such as Meals on Wheels, provide reasonably priced meals delivered to the home. A housekeeper/cook and cooking classes are usually out of the budget for most low-income people. An assisted living facility is usually not covered by Medicare or insurance and can be expensive.

Refer to: Subdomain–Resources for the Uninsured or Underinsured.

15. Answer: B

Rationale: The first step is to identify the barriers to compliance with the member in order to develop a plan to overcome the barriers. For example, a client who is non-compliant with his follow-up visits due to transportation issues can be referred to community resources for transportation.

Refer to: Subdomain–Management of Client With Acute and Chronic Illness.

16. Answer: B

Rationale: The case manager should encourage the patient to explore her feelings without judgment, in a supportive environment.

Refer to: Subdomain–Psychosocial Aspects of Chronic Illness and Disability.

17. Answer: C

Rationale: When the client's cultural beliefs conflict with the treatment plan, the case manager should attempt to adjust the treatment plan to work within the cultural limits. If this is not possible, the case manager must educate the client on the possible effects of not complying with the treatment plan. They should be done respectfully without coercing the client.

Refer to: Subdomain–Multicultural, Spiritual, and Religious Factors.

18. Answer: C

Rationale: 5 Stages of Change

1. In the pre-contemplation stage, the individual does not intend to take action in the foreseeable future.

2. In the contemplation stage, the individual considers a change in the next six months but has not committed to it. He may be open to information on the benefits of change and how to successfully do so.

3. In the preparation stage, the client actively plans to make changes within the next month and may have taken small steps toward change.

4. Action is the stage when the individual has successfully made a change and has sustained it for less than six months.

5. Maintenance is when the individual has sustained the change for 6 months or more.

Refer to: Subdomain–Behavioral Change Theories and Stages.

Chapter Five:
Quality and Outcomes
Evaluations and Measurements

Quality and Outcomes Evaluation and Measurements comprise 19% of the exam with between 27 and 31 questions on this topic.

****

Everyone—from policymakers to payers to accrediting bodies—is requiring the healthcare industry to focus on quantifiable outcomes. With the recent trend of healthcare reimbursement being tied to quantifiable outcomes, there is a heightened focus on quality, efficiency, safety, and value in healthcare.

Case managers are in a position to shine in this environment, by means of their opportunities to directly affect outcomes from patient admission through discharge and beyond. In many cases, case managers work hand in hand with Quality department personnel as the daily "eyes and ears" of a strong Quality Improvement plan.

Case managers must be familiar with quality and outcome measures, the impact these measures have on their setting, and must understand their role in ensuring organizations meet them.

<<<< >>>>

Quality and Performance Improvement Concepts

Quality improvement is a systematic, data-driven effort to measure and improve client services and the quality of healthcare services provided. It is accomplished by monitoring, correcting, and preventing quality deficiencies and noncompliance with the standards of care. It is not intended to attribute blame, but rather to discover where errors are occurring and to develop systems to prevent errors.

Performance improvement focuses on the healthcare organization's functions and processes and how these affect the ability to reach desired outcomes and meet the client's needs. Both quality improvement and performance improvement can be prospective or retrospective, and aim to improve how things are done.

There are several measurements for performance improvement, including:

1. Process
2. Structure
3. Outcomes

Measures of Process examine what is actually done in giving and receiving care and how well clinical guidelines are followed.

For example:
- Percentage of clients screened for colon cancer
- Percentage of patients with diabetes given regular foot care
- Percentage of children who are vaccinated
- Percentage of heart patients who receive beta-blockers in the hospital

Measures of Structure assess the capacity of a healthcare organization to provide services to individual patients or a community, and for managed care organizations, to ensure they have network providers in place to meet members' needs. For example:

- Accreditation status
- Staffing ratios
- Board-certified providers
- Access to specific technologies or units (e.g., MRI, burn unit)

Measures of Outcomes examine the health status of the patient as a result of healthcare. For example:

- Adherence rates
- Control of blood pressure
- Acceptable HgA1c levels
- Mortality

The Intersection of Quality and Case Management

The Case Management Society of America (CMSA) defines case management as a collaborative process of assessment, planning, facilitation, care coordination, evaluation, and advocacy for options and services to meet an individual's and family's comprehensive health needs through communication and available resources to promote quality, cost-effective outcomes. (CMSA, 2020).

Case management programs should maintain a quality management function to show the value case management brings to both the client and the healthcare organization. The case management program could be eliminated if it does not demonstrate the value it brings.

Case management programs should promote objective monitoring and evaluation of the case management services rendered. The program should also provide written documentation of the quality or performance improvement goals, as well as strategies to monitor and evaluate the case management quality. Program requirements are often determined by the accrediting organization of the setting.

For example, acute care facilities are bound by the Center for Medicare and Medicaid Conditions of Participation (CoP). These Conditions of Participation were created and are evaluated annually to ensure a minimum expectation for health and safety standards, which ultimately leads to improving the quality of care and protecting beneficiaries of these programs. Adherence to the CoP is mandatory for participation in both Medicare and Medicaid programs.

Similarly, managed care organizations can opt for accreditation by one of several entities. Program requirements and quality improvement expectations are governed by the standards put forth by these organizations. Again, the standards set the requirement for accreditation by the accreditor.

Data related to case management services and quality performance goals should be tracked, and steps should be taken to enhance areas identified as needing improvement. Healthcare's ability to accurately and meaningfully measure, evaluate and re-evaluate the outcomes and therefore, the quality of healthcare is essential to assessment and improvement. "Simply put, you cannot demonstrably improve what you cannot measure; and to measure, you need good data—data that is fair, accurate, and robust. Good data allows you not only to assess the quality of care, but also to measure the effect of the quality improvement intervention. Continuous quality improvement depends on determining what improves quality and what doesn't by using good data to continually assess and reassess healthcare quality" (Schmidt, 2012). Case Management is well positioned to use data to drive process improvement across the continuum of care.

The professional case manager provides valuable input and insight into driving process improvement and we must never lose sight of that. We all know of the anecdotal "stories from the front" that identify issues and opportunities, however, without the data to support these stories; making the case for a process improvement falls flat. Qualitative data, in the form of anecdotal information (or stories), helps to identify potential issues. Quantitative data, collected based on those stories, highlights the severity of the issues and provides insight into potential solutions. Leveraging data does not only reinforce the process of care provision but also fosters better patient outcomes and overall improvement of health. Case management documentation is vital to achieving these goals.

Quality Indicators and Applications

Quality indicators are defined as objective and quantitative measures of the structures, processes, or outcomes of care. Indicators provide a quantitative starting point for clinicians, organizations, and planners who strive to achieve improvement in care and the processes by which patient care is provided.

Indicators themselves do not provide definitive answers but they do suggest good quality care or potential problems.

The following are types of quality indicators and examples of what they measure.

Clinical - Pain management, level of function, rehospitalization/ readmissions, hospital-acquired conditions, avoiding hospitalization in favor of appropriate lower levels of care, rates of morbidity, mortality, and complications

Financial – Cost per case, cost per service, cost per day, length of stay, avoidable or unreimbursed days, denials (by reason for denial; administrative, medical necessity, timely filing, failure to notify)

Productivity – Wait time for appointment, length of time client spends in transplant evaluation before being presented to the Medical Review Board, length of stay

Utilization – Cesarean section delivery rate, incidental appendectomy in the elderly, hysterectomy rate, appropriate level of care, appropriate level of service

Quality – Decubitus ulcer rate, foreign body left in during a procedure, hospital-acquired infection

Client experience – Satisfaction, comfort, willingness to recommend

Monitoring healthcare quality is impossible without the use of quality indicators. They create the basis for quality improvement and prioritization in the healthcare system by identifying potential quality concerns, identifying areas requiring further investigation, and tracking changes over time. Measuring and monitoring of quality indicators can serve many purposes, including:

- Documenting quality of care

- Comparing care over time

- Comparing care between places (e.g., geographical, hospital); also referred to as "benchmarking"

- Supporting accountability, such as accreditation and/or regulation

- Supporting quality improvement projects

The information needed to assess quality indicators can be acquired by systematic or non-systematic methods. Ideally, systematic methods should be based on scientific evidence, but this type of evidence is not available for many areas of healthcare. In these cases, quality indicators can be based on a combination of evidence and the professional opinion and experience of clinicians.

One popular method for obtaining professional opinions for quality indicators is the Delphi technique, a structured process that uses a series of questionnaires, known as rounds, to gather information. Rounds are held until a group consensus is reached. A primary benefit of the Delphi technique is that a large number of professionals in various locations with diverse scopes of expertise can be included.

Benchmarking aids a healthcare organization to assess how the entity performs against its peers and where improvement might be pursued. In a 2018 survey performed by Health Catalyst, 72% of healthcare executives said "to identify and prioritize improvement opportunities, benchmarks are important or extremely important" (Health Catalyst, 2018). Furthermore, benchmarks give organizations a target or goal to work towards when in unfamiliar territory or working on new initiatives.

Non-systematic methods are quick and simple, but because they are not evidence-based, the resulting indicators may be less credible than those developed using systematic methods. Even so, indicators developed using non-systematic methods, such as case studies, can be useful. Because these methods are easier to perform than systematic methods, they allow for quicker application.

Quality indicators measure aspects of care, but measuring itself does not improve quality or outcomes. Measuring may identify a problem, so quality improvement can be applied.

Quality Improvement Strategies

In general, quality improvement methods use the Plan-Do-Study-Act (PDSA) approach. Two other popular quality improvement techniques used in healthcare are Six Sigma and Lean. The techniques are described below.

Plan-Do-Study-Act approach

As defined by the Institute for Healthcare Improvement, PDSA is "the scientific method, used in action oriented learning," testing changes in real life settings. The PDSA model asks 3 questions:

1. What are we trying to accomplish? The team identifies the issue and sets goals that are time-specific and measurable.

2. How will we know that the change is an improvement? The team uses data to determine if the change actually affects improvement. Anecdotal information is not reliable for this step. Measurable is key to demonstrating results.

3. What change can we make that will result in improvement? Be open to suggestions from all stakeholders.

In the PDSA approach, the Plan stage identifies a process that has yielded less than ideal outcomes. The Do stage measures key performance attributes.

Study devises a new approach, and Act integrates the redesigned approach into the process. Each episode is referred to as a "cycle." PDSA cycles can test change on a small scale (pilot), evaluate the findings, and refine the change as needed as the change is implemented on a wider scale.

***For more information on PDSA methodology, please refer to the Institute for Healthcare Improvement at http://www.ihi.org/resources/Pages/HowtoImprove/ScienceofImprovementHowtoImprove.aspx

Six Sigma approach

Six Sigma focuses on eliminating defects; defects in products, process, or practice. Six Sigma for Healthcare can be used to improve patient safety via the elimination of errors in process or practice. These projects can range from prescribing errors to improving nurse shift change assignments to improving patient flow. Using a 5-step approach to process improvement, known by the acronym DMAIC: define, measure, analyze, improve, and control.

Define – In the Define step, the goal and scope of the project are identified (e.g., decreasing hospital length of stay (LOS) after hip replacement).

Measure – Measure involves collecting available data for the process to develop a baseline. In this step, the team also identifies all interrelated business processes to find areas of possible performance enhancement (e.g., determining current LOS for hip replacements, and listing all disciplines involved with the patient).

Analyze – The objective of the third step, Analyze, is to reveal the root cause of inefficiencies, and to determine solutions to overcome these inefficiencies. Group discussions and analysis of the data collected in the Measure step will reveal where changes can provide the most effective results (e.g., Physical Therapy and Occupational Therapy are not available over the weekend, resulting in a delay of treatment; availability of these disciplines over the weekend will eliminate this delay).

Improve – The fourth step, Improve, develops and implements methods to address the process deficiencies uncovered during analysis. By the end of this phase, a test run of the change is completed and feedback is analyzed (e.g., PT and OT are available on the weekend; LOS is reevaluated).

Control – In the Control stage, metrics are developed to assess the success of the implemented changes. If adjustments must be made, the cycle will continue. Alternatively, the new changes may be made permanent, and the project is complete.

Lean approach

The Lean approach to quality improvement emphasizes reducing waste to increase value. Waste is identified as one of 8 areas, using the acronym DOWNTIME.

D: Defects

O: Overproduction

W: Waiting

N: Non-utilized talent

T: Transportation

I: Inventory

M: Motion

E: Extra-processing

Focus is placed on the customers, including patients, payers, providers, and regulatory bodies, to determine what they consider valuable. Lean provides tools for analyzing process flow and delay times to distinguish "value-added" work from "non-value-added" work. When the non-value-added work (or "waste") is identified, it is eliminated. The elimination of waste can increase value, decrease costs, and create a better customer experience.

***For more information on LEAN, please refer to https://asq.org/quality-resources/lean

Kaizen

Lean and Six Sigma can be combined in a "Kaizen" event, merging both philosophies. Kaizen means continuous improvement. Kaizen events are team events where a process is taken apart, process mapped, and opportunities for improvement identified as a team exercise, allowing for input from all stakeholders along the way. Kaizen activities are a continuous cycle with seven phases:

1. Identify an opportunity: what is the issue?

2. Analyze the process: deconstruct and map the process, identifying potential gaps.

3. Develop an optimal solution: what is the goal? How can we get there? Create a roadmap.

4. Implement the solution: implement the roadmap.

5. Study the results: what happened? Success, continued challenges, fix the challenges, re-implement until success achieved.

6. Standardize the solution: implement across all like units.

7. Plan for the future: how do we make sure this becomes part of the culture and what do we do to avoid deviations? How often do we evaluate for updates?

***For more information on Kaizen, please refer to https://www.isixsigma.com/methodology/kaizen/kaizen-six-sigma-ensures-continuous-improvement/

Accreditation Standards and Requirements

Accreditation is usually a voluntary process, provided by an external organization, in which trained peer reviewers evaluate a healthcare organization's compliance with nationally accepted standards, as well as the accrediting body's pre-established performance standards. Although accreditation is technically voluntary, it is often required to be eligible to receive reimbursement from Medicare, Medicaid, and many third-party payers. Accreditation is also often required by local, state, or federal regulations.

Accreditation is regarded as one of the key benchmarks for measuring the quality of an organization. It identifies the organization as credible and reputable, dedicated to ongoing and continuous compliance with the highest standard of quality. There is consistent evidence that accreditation significantly improves the process of care provided by healthcare services and improves clinical outcomes.

Preparing for accreditation provides a healthcare organization the opportunity to improve the quality of care they provide to patients by establishing, reviewing, and revising standards, measuring performance, and providing education. It is a chance for the organization to identify its strengths and its opportunities for improvement.

An accrediting body might review the organizational structure, policies and procedures, quality outcomes, performance improvement, patients' rights, professional improvement, leadership, fiscal operations, and clinical records, as well as compliance with federal, state, and local laws.

There are numerous accrediting bodies covering the various healthcare industries, including but not limited to:

- Commission on Accreditation of Rehabilitation Facilities (CARF)
- URAC
- National Committee for Quality Assurance (NCQA)
- Joint Commission

They have their own standards and requirements for awarding accreditation based on their corner of the healthcare industry, but the objective is always to ensure consumer protection by requiring safe, quality care.

Sources of Quality Indicators

The next few pages are devoted to some of the accrediting bodies and sources of quality indicators case managers should be familiar with. A general overview is given for each, with examples when appropriate. For more information or a complete list of standards, links are provided on our website CCMcertificationMadeEasy.com. It is recommended to look up any terminology that is not understood for more details.

CARF

The Commission on Accreditation of Rehabilitation Facilities (CARF) is an independent, non-profit accreditor of health and human services. CARF's standards focus on improved service outcomes, client satisfaction, and quality service delivery. Each set of standards is developed with the input of providers, consumers, payers, and other experts from around the world. Each year, CARF updates its standards to ensure they are relevant and guide excellent service.

CARF provides accreditation in the following areas:

- Medical rehabilitation
- Durable medical equipment, prosthetics, orthotics, and supplies
- Aging services
- Behavioral health, including opioid treatment programs
- Employment and community services
- Child and youth services
- Business and services management networks

***Additional information can be found on CARF's website at http://www.carf.org/Accreditation/

URAC

URAC, formerly known as the Utilization Review Accreditation Commission, accredits over 20 types of healthcare organizations, including Accountable

Care, Case Management, Community Pharmacy, Disease Management, and Health Plan. URAC accreditation standards and requirements vary based on the type of organization being accredited.

As a credentialing body for case management, URAC believes that effective case management puts the consumer at the center of all healthcare decisions, and that this is essential to ensuring consumers get the right care, in the right setting, at the right time. URAC's Case Management accreditation allows case management standards to be applied across all healthcare settings, such as medical and social case management, behavioral health providers, hospital case management, disability and workers' compensation case management, and emerging practices. URAC has 40 CORE standards in 14 areas that apply to case management organizations.

URAC's case management standards cover:

- Organizational structure
- Policies and procedures
- Regulatory compliance
- Departmental coordination
- Oversight of delegated functions
- Review of marketing and sales material
- Business relationships: written business agreements, client satisfaction
- Information management: business continuity, information confidentiality and security, confidentiality of individually identifiable health information
- Quality management: quality management program, resources, and requirements; quality management committee, documentation, projects, project requirements, and consumer organizations
- Staff qualifications
- Staff management: training programs, operational tools and support, assessment programs

- Clinical staff credentialing and oversight roles
- Healthcare system coordination
- Consumer protection and empowerment: consumer rights and responsibilities, safety mechanisms, satisfaction, and health literacy

***Additional information can be found on URAC's website at https://www.urac.org/ accreditation-and-measurement/accreditation-and-measurement

NCQA

The National Committee for Quality Assurance (NCQA) provides accreditation for healthcare organizations and managed care organizations. They also sponsor, support, and maintain a collection of standardized performance measures known as the Healthcare Effectiveness Data and Information Set (HEDIS). The information from HEDIS helps employers and other purchasers evaluate health plan operations.

The case management accreditation provided by the NCQA is based on comprehensive and evidence-based guidelines, and it is dedicated to quality improvement. The core of the accreditation program is care coordination, patient-centeredness, and quality of care. It can be used for case management programs in provider, payer, population health, or community-based organizations.

NCQA's Case Management Accreditation:

- Directly addresses how case management services are delivered, not just the organization's internal administrative processes.
- Gets to the essence of care coordination and quality of care.
- Is designed for a wide variety of organizations. It is appropriate for health plans, providers, population health management organizations, and community-based case management organizations.
- Focuses on ensuring the organization has a process for safe transitions.

The standards address how case management programs:

- Identify people in need of case management services.
- Target the right services to clients and monitor their care and needs over time.
- Develop personalized, patient-centered care plans.
- Monitor clients to ensure care plan goals are reached and make adjustments as needed.
- Manage communication among providers and share information effectively as people move between care settings, especially when they transition from institutional settings.
- Build in consumer protections to ensure people have access to knowledgeable, well-qualified case management staff.
- Keep personal health information safe and secure.

HEDIS

Healthcare Effectiveness Data and Information Set (HEDIS) consists of more than 90 measures in six healthcare domains of care:

1. Effectiveness of care: includes immunization status, screenings for cancers, such as breast, colorectal and cervical, condition management strategies and education

2. Access/Availability of care: access to all levels and specialties of care

3. Experience of care: patient satisfaction with service and care

4. Utilization and Risk Adjusted Utilization: procedure frequency, antibiotic stewardship, infection rates, readmissions, emergency department use versus doctor office visits

5. Health Plan Descriptive Information

6. Measures Collected Using Electronic Clinical Data Systems: depression screenings, unhealthy alcohol use, and adult immunizations

NCQA standards also call for case management program staff to stay up to date on the latest evidence and case management techniques and work toward continuous improvement in patient outcomes and satisfaction.

***Additional information on NCQA's case management accreditation can be found at https://www.ncqa.org/programs/health-plans/case-management-cm/

The Joint Commission

The Joint Commission (TJC) offers accreditation programs for a variety of healthcare settings, such as; Ambulatory Care, Behavioral Health, Home Care, Hospital, Laboratory Services, and Nursing Care Centers.

Certification programs are offered for condition/disease management programs including Palliative Care, Total Hip and Knee Replacement, Cardiac diagnoses, and Stroke.

The Primary Care Medical Home & Integrated Care certifications focus on healthcare models with a patient-centered care philosophy, providing comprehensive care across settings, using clinical integration, data-sharing, and shared performance improvement processes.

***Additional information on The Joint Commission's Accreditation and Certification programs can be found at https://www.jointcommission.org/accreditation-and-certification/#8716301c6b2a4a6490d0bad4862bfa0a

Other Important Healthcare Quality Organizations

NQF

The National Quality Forum (NQF) is a not-for-profit, nonpartisan, membership-based organization whose mission is to improve the quality of healthcare. NQF promotes consensus among a wide variety of stakeholders from both the public and private sector, around specific standards that can be used to measure and publicly report healthcare quality.

NQF has endorsed performance measures to quantify healthcare processes, outcomes, patient perceptions, and organizational structures or systems that provide high-quality care. Once a measure is endorsed by NQF, it can be used by hospitals, healthcare systems, and government agencies like the Centers for Medicare & Medicaid Services, for public reporting and quality improvement.

NQF performance measures:

- Bring together working groups to foster quality improvement in both public and private sectors
- Endorse consensus standards for performance measurement
- Ensure that consistent, high-quality performance information is publicly available
- Seek real-time feedback to ensure measures are meaningful and accurate

NQF-endorsed measures are evidence-based. Together with the delivery of care and payment reform, they help:

- Make patient care safer
- Improve maternity care
- Achieve better health outcomes
- Strengthen chronic care management
- Hold down healthcare costs

***More information on NQF can be found at http://www.qualityforum.org/Measures_ Reports_Tools.aspx

CMS

Quality Improvement Organizations/ Quality Improvement Networks of the Centers for Medicare & Medicaid Services

The Centers for Medicare & Medicaid Services (CMS) is a federal agency within the U.S. Department of Health and Human Services. CMS contracts with agencies to manage the two-fold initiative of Quality Improvement Organizations (QIOs) and Quality Innovation Networks (QIN), which work under the direction of CMS; they are a group of health quality experts, clinicians, and consumers, organized to improve the care delivered to people covered by Medicare. By law, the mission of the QIO/QIN Program is to improve the effectiveness, efficiency, economy, and quality of services delivered to Medicare beneficiaries. Each side is separate from the other but has a common goal to improve the quality of services/care provided to Medicare beneficiaries.

QIO

BFCC-QIOs (Beneficiary and Family Centered Care QIO) do this by analyzing data and patient records to identify areas for improvements in care. They also ensure patients' voices are heard by addressing individual complaints.

CMS identifies the core functions of the QIO Program as:

- Improving quality of care for beneficiaries
- Protecting the integrity of the Medicare Trust Fund by ensuring that Medicare pays only for services and goods that are reasonable and necessary, and that are provided in the most appropriate setting
- Protecting beneficiaries by expeditiously addressing individual complaints, such as beneficiary complaints; provider-based notice appeals; violations of the Emergency Medical Treatment and Labor Act (EMTALA); and other related responsibilities as articulated in QIO-related law
- Providing Health Care Navigation services

The CMS uses Clinical Quality Measures, or CQMs, to ensure that healthcare systems deliver effective, safe, efficient, patient-centered, equitable, and timely care. Clinical quality measures track the quality of healthcare services provided. They examine providers' ability to deliver high-quality care or relate to long-term goals for quality healthcare.

CQMs measure many aspects of patient care, including:

- Health outcomes
- Clinical processes
- Patient safety
- Efficient use of healthcare resources
- Care coordination
- Patient engagements
- Population and public health
- Adherence to clinical guidelines

QIN-QIO

The Quality Innovation Network-Quality Improvement Organization (QIN-QIO) is made up of twelve regional contractors that work with providers, community partners, beneficiaries, and caregivers on data-driven quality improvement initiatives designed to improve the quality of healthcare for people with specific conditions or address specific gaps in healthcare for Medicare beneficiaries.

QIN-QIO initiatives provide access to valuable resources, including evidence-based improvement strategies that are aligned with other major health quality initiatives. QIN-QIO shares knowledge on critical healthcare quality and safety issues while disseminating real-world best practices for implementation locally or regionally. Healthcare entities such as hospitals, hospital systems, practice groups, and other healthcare providers, can partner with the QIO Program to make a difference in their own communities while contributing to national health quality goals that benefit all Americans.

The QIN-QIO Program can also help healthcare entities understand what is involved in different national quality initiatives and how they all work together to improve healthcare quality, accessibility, and affordability. As one of the largest federal programs dedicated to improving health quality at the local level, the

QIN-QIO programs help healthcare providers to deliver person-centered, safer, and more effective care in their communities.

QIN-QIO has national, regional, and local level information and projects focused on three major areas:

1. Improving population health

    a. Reducing cardiac care, diabetes care disparities

    b. Stroke prevention

    c. Improving adult immunization rates

    d. Improving the identification of depression and ETOH use in primary care and care transitions for behavioral health

2. Improving quality within the healthcare system

    a. Antibiotic stewardship programs

    b. Decreasing healthcare acquired conditions in nursing homes

    c. Promoting effective care coordination and communication

    d. Increasing medication safety

3. Reducing the cost of care

    a. Providing technical assistance on participation in Quality Payment Program (QPP)

    b. Assist in data analysis, interpretation to drive quality improvements

    c. Facilitates networking for support and best practice sharing

***For more information on the QIN-QIO, please refer to: https://qioprogram.org/health-care-providers

Core Measures of the Centers for Medicare & Medicaid Services

CMS also identifies a set of care standards known as Core Measures. Core Measures are standards that have been shown through scientific evidence to improve patient outcomes, and they set the standard for care provided to patients while in the hospital.

As the healthcare system moves toward value-based reimbursement models, providers are required to report multiple quality measures to many different entities. To address this issue, CMS created the Core Quality Measures Collaborative, where CMS, commercial plans, Medicare and Medicaid managed plans, NQF, physicians, care provider organizations, and consumers work together to identify core sets of quality measures. The Core Quality Measures Collaborative established agreed-upon core measure sets that are coordinated across both government and commercial payers. Seven core measure sets were created and can be viewed in the table on the following page.

The goals of the Core Measures are quality-focused; promoting evidence-based practices and validated measurements that help consumers in decision making, provide an "even playing field" for measurement and evaluation across the healthcare environment, and provide a basis for value-based purchasing and payment initiatives.

***More information on Core Measures and links to complete lists can be found at
https://www.cms.gov/Medicare/Quality-Initiatives-Patient-Assessment-Instruments/ QualityMeasures/Core-Measures.html

Core Measure	Examples of Items Measured
Cardiology	• Therapy with aspirin, P2Y12 inhibitor, and statin at discharge following PCI in eligible patients • Primary PCI received within 90 minutes of hospital arrival
Accountable Care Organizations, Patient Centered Medical Homes, and Primary Care	• Persistent beta blocker treatment after a heart attack • Comprehensive diabetes care: eye exam, hemoglobin A1c (HbA1c) testing, foot exam, medical attention for nephropathy • Cervical cancer screening
Gastroenterology	• Age appropriate screening colonoscopy • Screening for Hepatocellular Carcinoma (HCC) in patients with Hepatitis C • One-time screening for Hepatitis C Virus (HCV) for patients at risk
HIV and Hepatitis C	• Pneumocystis jiroveci pneumonia (PCP) prophylaxis for HIV patients • HIV viral load suppression • One-time screening for Hepatitis C Virus (HCV) for patients at risk
Medical Oncology	• Patients with breast cancer and negative or undocumented human epidermal growth factor receptor 2 (HER2) status who are spared treatment with trastuzumab • Radical prostatectomy pathology reporting • Proportion of members receiving chemotherapy in the last 14 days of life
Obstetrics and Gynecology	• Breast cancer and cervical cancer screening • Exclusive breast milk feeding • Elective delivery and cesarean section rate
Orthopedics	• Hospital-level risk-standardized complication rate (RSCR) following elective primary total hip arthroplasty (THA) and/or total knee arthroplasty (TKA) • Patient experience with surgical care based on the Consumer Assessment of Healthcare Providers and Systems (CAHPS) Surgical Care Survey

AHRQ

The Agency for Healthcare Research and Quality (AHRQ) is part of the U.S. Department of Health and Human Services. The agency publishes and disseminates national clinical practice guidelines. Its mission is to produce evidence to make healthcare safer, higher quality, and more accessible, equitable, and affordable. The data used to measure performance include administrative data such as billing or claims data, medical record information, patient-derived data such as surveys, confidential reports from providers, and direct observation.

The Quality Indicators (QIs) established and maintained by the AHRQ are evidence-based and can be used to identify variations in the quality of care provided on both an inpatient and outpatient basis. The QIs consist of four models measuring various aspects of quality: Prevention Quality Indicators (PQIs), Inpatient Quality Indicators (IQIs), Patient Safety Indicators (PSIs), and Pediatric Indicators (PDIs).

Prevention Quality Indicators (PQIs) – Identifies conditions where good outpatient care can potentially prevent the need for hospitalization, or in which early intervention can prevent complications or an increase in disease severity.

Examples of PQIs are:
- Hypertension admission rate
- Congestive heart failure admission rate
- Low birth weight rate
- Angina admission without procedure
- Uncontrolled diabetes admission rate

Inpatient Quality Indicators (IQIs) – Indicators reflecting the quality of care inside hospitals, including inpatient mortality; the utilization of procedures that are questionably misused, overused, or underused; and procedure volume where higher volume is associated with lower mortality.

Examples of the mortality indicators for inpatient surgical procedures include:

- Abdominal aortic aneurysm (AAA) repair mortality rate
- Coronary artery bypass graft (CABG) mortality rate
- Hip replacement mortality rate

Examples of the mortality indicators for inpatient medical conditions include:

- Acute myocardial infarction (AMI) mortality rate
- Congestive heart failure mortality rate
- Hip fracture mortality rate
- Pneumonia mortality rate

Examples of the procedure utilization indicators include:

- Primary cesarean delivery rate
- Vaginal birth after cesarean (VBAC) rate
- Laparoscopic cholecystectomy rate

Examples of the IQIs that focus on volume include:

- Pancreatic resection volume
- Abdominal aortic aneurysm (AAA) repair volume
- Coronary artery bypass graft (CABG) volume
- Carotid endarterectomy (CEA) volume

Patient Safety Indicators (PSIs) – Potentially preventable instances of complications and other iatrogenic events resulting from exposure to the healthcare system. There are currently 27 PSIs covering two levels: the provider level (within a hospital) and the area level (within a metropolitan service area or county).

Examples of provider-level PSIs include:

- Postoperative pulmonary embolism or deep vein thrombosis
- Postoperative respiratory failure
- Postoperative hemorrhage or hematoma
- Decubitus ulcer

- Foreign body left in during procedure
- Birth trauma – injury to neonate
- Obstetric trauma – cesarean section delivery
- Complications of anesthesia
- Transfusion reaction (AB/Rh)

Examples of the area-level PSIs include:

- Foreign body left in during procedure
- Selected infections due to medical care
- Postoperative wound dehiscence in abdominopelvic surgical patients
- Accidental puncture or laceration
- Transfusion reaction
- Postoperative hemorrhage or hematoma

Pediatric Quality Indicators (PDIs) – These indicators reflect the quality of care for neonates and children younger than 17 inside the hospital and identify potentially avoidable hospitalizations among children. There are currently 13 provider-level PDIs and 5 area-level PDIs

Examples of provider-level PDIs include:

- Foreign body left in during procedure
- Iatrogenic pneumothorax in neonates
- Postoperative hemorrhage or hematoma
- Postoperative sepsis
- Transfusion reaction

Examples of area-level PDIs are:

- Asthma admission rate
- Perforated appendix admission rate
- Urinary tract infection admission rate

In addition to the Quality Indicators, AHRQ also maintains the Healthcare Cost and Utilization Project (HCUP); a comprehensive source of hospital data; including ambulatory surgery, emergency department visits, and inpatient stays. Data available includes diagnoses, procedures, demographics, discharge status, and charges, regardless of payer. This data can be used for benchmarking, research, policy development and evaluation of access to healthcare, patient outcomes, and cost/quality of care. The information is available through any one of seven databases:

1. National (Nationwide) Inpatient Sample (NIS)

2. Kids' Inpatient Database (KID)

3. Nationwide Emergency Department Sample (NEDS)

4. Nationwide Readmissions Database

5. State Inpatient Database (SID)

6. State Ambulatory Surgery and Services Databases (SASD)

7. State Emergency Department Databases (SEDD)

***More information on AHRQ and links to complete lists of their QIs can be found at http://www.ncbi.nlm.nih.gov/books/NBK2664/

National Quality Strategy (NQS)

The National Quality Strategy (NQS) was first published in March 2011 as the National Strategy for Quality Improvement in Health Care, and is led by the AHRQ. Developed with input from stakeholders representing all members of the care continuum and general public, the NQS is defined by a "3-6-9 strategy"; a set of "three overarching gains" building on IHI's Triple Aim, six priorities of common health concerns and nine "levers" to align business/organizational functions and drive quality improvement (AHRQ, 2017).

Improving health and healthcare quality can occur only if all stakeholders—individuals, family members, payers, providers, employers, and communities—make it a priority.

Three Overarching Gains

Used to provide guidance/set goals at all levels in the improvement of health and the quality of healthcare.

1. Better Care: Improving health care quality with a focus on patient-centered, reliable, accessible, and safe

2. Healthy People/Healthy Communities: Population health initiatives to address behavioral, social, and environmental determinants of health

3. Affordable Care: Reduce the cost of quality health care for all stakeholders

Six Priorities

1. Making care safer by reducing harm.

2. Increasing patient/family engagement as "partners in their care."

3. Promoting effective communication and coordination of care.

4. Promoting the most effective prevention and treatment practices for the leading causes of mortality.

5. Promotion of wide use of best practices in communities to enable healthy living.

6. Increasing access to quality care through affordability for all by developing and spreading new/innovative health care delivery models.

Nine Levers

Core business functions, resources, and/or actions that stakeholders use to align with NQS. Conscious connection to NQS strategies of levers already in place can help to align strategies more fully.

1. Measurement and Feedback

2. Public Reporting

3. Learning and Technical Assistance

4. Certification, Accreditation, and Regulation

5. Consumer Incentives and Benefit Designs

6. Payment

7. Health Information Technology

8. Innovation and Diffusion

9. Workforce Development

The NQS ultimately supports the sharing of best practices in health and healthcare quality improvement at the national, state, and local levels, and promotes collaboration across the care continuum at all levels (AHRQ, 2017).

***Stakeholder toolkits, FAQs and other resources are available at https://www.ahrq.gov/workingforquality/reports/progress.html

Data Interpretation and Reporting

When interpreting data, validity and reliability must be taken into consideration. Validity refers to the meaningfulness of the data being measured; that is, is it measuring what it is intended to measure. Reliability refers to the accuracy. The case manager must ensure that data gathered is reliable by avoiding bias.

After data is collected, it must be interpreted. This is the process of assigning meaning to information collected and determining the conclusions, significance, and implications of the findings. It is important once again to avoid any bias while interpreting the data. Information obtained during the data collection and interpretation is then reported.

As care coordinators, case managers must be able to show that the interventions implemented changed the patient's outcome. This information is shown in case management reports.

Several of the reports case managers use include:

- Patient satisfaction surveys (HCAHPS)
- Patient care reports
- Quality improvement
- Cost-benefit of case management services
- Justification to continue intervention
- Demonstrating lack of results with current intervention to justify approving more costly intervention

Hospital Consumer Assessment of Healthcare Providers and Systems (HCAHPS)

HCAHPS (pronounced "H-caps"), also known as the CAHPS Hospital Survey, is a nationally standardized survey of patients' perspectives of their hospital experience. The survey was developed by Centers for Medicare and Medicaid Services (CMS) in partnership with Agency for Healthcare Research and Quality (AHRQ) and endorsed by National Quality Forum (NQF).

The results of this survey allow for an objective comparison of hospitals on topics that are important to consumers. These survey results are publicly reported, creating increased transparency of healthcare, as well as incentives for hospitals to improve the quality of care they provide.

The Deficit Reduction Act of 2005 and the Affordable Care Act of 2010 impacted HCAHPS measurements. In accordance with the Deficit Reduction Act, hospitals subject to the Inpatient Prospective Payment System (IPPS) annual payment update provisions must collect and submit HCAHPS data in order to receive their full IPPS annual payment update. IPPS hospitals that fail to publicly report the required quality measures, which include the HCAHPS survey, may receive a reduced payment. The Affordable Care Act includes HCAHPS among the measures used to calculate value-based incentive payments in the Hospital Value-Based Purchasing program.

Patient Care Reports

Patient Care Reports are important, as this is where case managers document the value of case management involvement. By recording the patient's condition prior to case management, the goals of case management, the patient's current condition relative to the goals, and case management interventions, case managers are able to demonstrate the value they bring.

Example: At case opening, client was unclear regarding his diagnosis. Case manager educated client regarding diagnosis. Client has a better understanding of his diagnosis and is now able to verbalize that understanding.

The frequency of patient reports may vary but should always be done at case closure. Patient Care Reports may include:
- Justification for case management involvement, such as the diagnosis
- Desired outcomes and goals of case management
- Progress toward the outcomes
- Cost of care with case management intervention
- Cost of care without case management intervention
- Cost savings due to case management intervention

Quality Improvement (QI) Reports

Items included in Quality Improvement reports include:
- Indicator being measured
- Case management intervention
- Measurement used to evaluate response to intervention
- Improvement in quality directly related to case management intervention

QI reports summarize the results of the program elements over defined time periods (month, quarter, year) to demonstrate movement towards/away from goals established. These can be used to set goals for the upcoming time periods and identify any changes needed to the program if undesired results are demonstrated.

Cost-Benefit Reports

Cost-benefit reports provide a summary of case management interventions and document the overall costs of care/savings related to case management activities. Report items include:

- Diagnosis
- Summary of interventions
- Total time in case management
- Total cost without case management intervention
- Total cost with case management intervention
- Total cost savings

Justification of Continuation of Intervention

Some interventions need documentation of progress for continuation. In these cases, provide:

- Data from before the intervention was initiated
- Current data
- Goal of intervention

The following is an example for a patient receiving physical therapy:

- Data before initiating intervention: Ambulates 12 feet with wheeled walker and max assist.
- Current data: Ambulates 100 feet with straight cane and stand-by-assist.
- Goal of intervention: Ambulate 250 feet independently with the least restrictive assistive device.

Justify More Costly Intervention

When the current intervention does not produce the desired results, the case manager may alert the patient care team so an alternative plan of care can be proposed. If the cost of the new proposed plan of care is more expensive than the current plan of care, the case manager must document the rationale for the new plan. In this instance, she must provide:

- Prior data
- Data from current therapy/intervention showing minimal or no progress
- Duration of current intervention
- Cost of current intervention
- Proposed intervention
- Cost of proposed intervention
- Duration of proposed intervention
- Goal of proposed intervention

Cost-Benefit Analysis

A cost-benefit report formally documents monetary savings related to case management involvement. There are two types of savings: hard cost savings and soft cost savings.

Savings directly related to the case manager's actions are hard savings.

Examples of hard savings include:

- Transfer to a lower level of care
- Decrease in length of stay
- Negotiation to a lower rate for a service
- Change to an in-network provider

Soft cost savings are potential savings and are more difficult to measure than hard savings. Soft cost savings are costs avoided due to case management intervention. These may include:

- Avoided hospital readmission
- Prevention of medical complications
- Avoided ER visits

There is a formula to calculate cost savings. First, the cost of service with case management involvement (Actual Cost) is added to the cost of the case management service. This number is then subtracted from the cost of intervention without case management involvement (Potential Cost). The difference is the cost savings associated with case management involvement.

Cost savings = Potential Costs - (Actual Cost + Cost of Case Management)

In addition to documenting the effectiveness of case management, a cost-benefit report can be used to justify an Alternative Treatment Plan (ATP) or to compare costs of various treatment options.

Program Evaluation Methods

Case management programs must be evaluated for effectiveness in reaching the desired outcomes and goals. Formal evaluation is completed with outcomes data based on information documented and collected throughout the case management process. This gives insight into what is working and what needs modification. Two ways to evaluate the effectiveness of the case management program are to conduct surveys and to measure outcomes.

Case Management Satisfaction Survey

The patient can be surveyed for satisfaction at any point in a case management program, but all patients should be surveyed when their cases are closed.

The survey must be objective and evaluate the quality and effectiveness of the case management program. The results of the survey provide the patient's perspective and value of case management. To receive the most honest answers to the survey, the patient should be allowed to remain anonymous if desired.

Survey results have multiple purposes. They may be used for marketing purposes, or they can be used in quality assurance, showing where goals are met, and where training, process improvement, or other intervention needs to take place. Surveys may also give information on future specialized program development needs, leading to a formal needs assessment process. Other surveys that measure patient experience related to transitions of care include Care Transitions Measure (CTM-3), Patient Experience Questionnaire (PEQ) and the Medical Home Care Coordination Survey (MHCCS).

Case Management Outcomes

Clinical outcomes can be measured on groups of patients, such as patients with a specific disease or those requiring a particular service (e.g., hospitalization, home health), as well as individual cases. The outcomes measured depend on the setting in which case management is provided.

Examples of outcomes measured include:
- Percentage of patients readmitted to the hospital within 30 days
- Percentage of patients adherent to the treatment plan
- Average length of the hospital stay
- Percentage of clients who returned to work
- Percentage of clients who maintained hemoglobin A1C <9

Healthcare Analytics

The foundation of successful case management is in timely identification of the population most likely to need/benefit from case management services; such as populations of high risk or rising risk patients, higher social determinant of health impact, palliative or hospice care appropriate, or chronic condition management.

Health Risk Assessments, Predictive Modeling, and Adjusted Clinical Groups are tools to identify at-risk individuals who may benefit from case management services. The goal is to be proactive and provide services to prevent disease, complications, morbidity, mortality, and hospitalization, therefore reducing cost and improving quality of life.

Health Risk Assessment

The Health Risk Assessment (HRA) is a tool to assess a patient's health status, risk of negative health outcomes, and readiness to change certain behaviors. It is used to design a prevention plan, so the patient can take action to improve his or her health status and delay or prevent the onset of disease caused by reported at-risk behaviors.

There are three components to the HRA: the questionnaire, the risk calculation, and feedback. The questionnaire is a self-reported assessment that identifies health behaviors and risk factors known only to the patient, such as physical activity, dietary habits, and smoking. It may also include biometrics.

The table below shows information often included in the health risk assessment.

Category	Data
Demographic Data	Sex, age
Biometric Assessment	Height, weight, blood pressure, cholesterol, blood sugar
Lifestyle	Physical activity/exercise, smoking, alcohol intake, diet, seat belt use
Family Medical History	Cancer, diabetes, hypertension, hypercholesterolemia

To calculate the patient's risk, the healthcare provider reviews the questionnaire responses and biometric data, assesses the patient's health status, and evaluates the risk of developing certain diseases, disabilities, or injuries.

The third component to the HRA is the personalized feedback aimed at reducing risk factors. The healthcare provider suggests appropriate interventions and provides motivation to change unhealthy or at-risk behaviors.

HRAs do more than just evaluate risk for disease or disability, and they are sometimes referred to as health assessments or wellness profiles. HRAs are also used by employers for wellness programs, by fitness centers to screen members before using equipment, and by health insurance companies to identify individuals for disease management programs.

HRAs are also used during Medicaid enrollment to identify individuals with health problems that need immediate attention. The Affordable Care Act specifies that an HRA be part of the annual wellness visit for Medicare beneficiaries. The ACA also specifies that the HRA must identify chronic diseases, injury risk, modifiable risk factors, and urgent health needs.

Though the HRA is an important tool, there are some limitations and methodological concerns. The most obvious is that self-reporting can lead to inaccurate information, due to a patient's recall bias, lack of understanding of the questions, or reluctance to report socially unacceptable behaviors. In addition, factors such as language, culture, and literacy level can affect the results.

Predictive Modeling

Predictive modeling uses technology and statistical methods to analyze enormous amounts of data to predict outcomes for individual patients. A model can be simple or complex, but more complex models are more accurate in predicting outcomes. Most often the data comes from health plan claims and identifies patterns of physician, specialist, laboratory, pharmaceutical, ER, and hospital care.

The data is compiled, analyzed, and interpreted to proactively identify individuals who are in danger of developing a high-risk disease. The objective is to identify these high-risk individuals at the earliest opportunity and to begin implementing appropriate interventions. This allows for healthcare resources to be targeted toward those who can benefit most; supporting population health management, financial success, and better outcomes across the continuum of care.

Predictive modeling can be a critical tool in managing future resource consumption. It identifies individuals whose future medical expenses could be significant and would most benefit from appropriate education and intervention through a disease management or case management program. This improves the use of case management resources by focusing them on patients who need assistance. This early intervention also increases opportunities for success, decreases adverse outcomes, and brings costs under control.

Adjusted Clinical Group (ACG)

The Adjusted Clinical Group (ACG) System is a tool developed by Johns Hopkins University to assess risk. It uses the diagnostic and pharmaceutical code information from insurance claims and electronic medical records to measure morbidity in large populations based on disease patterns, age, and gender. It provides an accurate representation of the morbidity burden of populations, subgroups, or individual patients based on the overall picture, and not on individual diseases. This information is used to evaluate provider performance more accurately and fairly, set equitable payment rates, forecast healthcare utilization, and identify patients at high risk.

Unlike many traditional methods of identifying clients for case management, such as emergency department usage, hospitalization, or high dollar claims, the ACG Predictive Model identifies individuals who are likely to become high resource users. By focusing on developing patterns of morbidity, such as those seeing multiple providers and taking multiple prescriptions, it identifies individuals who can benefit from case management and care coordination earlier.

Evidence-Based Care Guidelines Related to Case Management

Evidence-based practice (EBP) is mandated for all healthcare professionals, regardless of their discipline. Each discipline creates their own evidence-based care library that is dedicated to and supports professionalism, patient safety, and quality of care. A profession is defined as including the following characteristics: a knowledge based on extensive, standardized education, service to a larger social system, code of ethics, autonomy, competence, commitment, and authority. The ongoing development of evidence-based practices for case management is imperative to validate what we do and how we do it. With so much information available, it is "mission critical" to be able to identify pertinent, quality EBP. Acquiring the skill set to perform "rapid critical appraisals" is essential to identify and utilize EBP effectively. The ability to critically appraise and interpret the quality of the purported evidence is vital to prevent "tabloid healthcare," based on hearsay, advertisement, and celebrity endorsement, from becoming mainstream rather than EBP.

Evidence-based practice is the process of applying the best available research when making decisions about healthcare. Numerous professionals analyze new research information and develop practice guidelines. The guidelines give the provider and the patient recommendations for screening, diagnostic workup, and treatment that are believed to provide the best outcome.

These guidelines are not meant to replace the clinical judgment of the individual provider or establish a standard of care. They are meant to be flexible and are only considered recommendations. Healthcare professionals who promote evidence-based guidelines use research evidence along with clinical expertise and patient preferences in providing care.

Treatment guidelines are similar to practice guidelines but focus on assisting providers in deciding on the most appropriate treatment for clinical conditions. Like practice guidelines, treatment guidelines are recommendations, not standards of care.

Standards of Care

Whereas guidelines are meant to be flexible, standards are a rigid set of criteria meant to be followed under any circumstances. These practices are medically necessary for the management of a clinical condition.

Clinical Pathway

A clinical pathway provides outcome-focused care within a certain timeline. Clinical pathways develop algorithms from evidence-based guidelines, standards of care, and protocols for common diagnoses, conditions, and procedures. These algorithms are used by a multidisciplinary care team in providing care to the patient. Clinical pathways standardize treatments, promote efficiency, and improve the continuity and coordination of care provided by all disciplines involved. This results in a greater quality of care and decreased costs.

Items addressed on the clinical pathway may include:

- Patient assessment and monitoring
- Tests and procedures
- Treatments
- Consultations
- Medications
- Activity
- Nutrition
- Education
- Targeted length of stay
- Outcome criteria
- Notification for deviations

BONUS

As a reminder, there are a lot of links in this chapter, and in this book. To get easy access to all of the links and resources mentioned for each chapter, make sure you visit

CCMcertificationMadeEasy.com

References

Agency for Healthcare and Quality. (2017, March). *About the national quality strategy.* https://www.ahrq.gov/workingforquality/about/index.html

Case Management Society of America. (n.d.). *What is a case manager?* https://www.cmsa.org/who-we-are/what-is-a-case-manager/

Commission for Case Management Certification. (2017). *Glossary of terms.* https://ccmcertification.org/get-certified/exam-study-materials/ccmc-glossary

Health Catalyst. (2018). Healthcare benchmarking. https://www.healthcatalyst.com/healthcare-benchmarking/

Institute of Healthcare Improvement. (n.d.). *Science of improving: How to improve.* http://www.ihi.org/resources/Pages/HowtoImprove/ScienceofImprovementHowtoImprove.aspx

Morley, C. (2019). Don't think case management data matters? Think again. CMSA Today, Issue 1, 2019.

National Institute on Drug Addiction. (2020, June 3). Types of treatment programs. Retrieved June 19, 2020, from https://www.drugabuse.gov/publications/principles-drug-addiction-treatment-research-based-guide-third-edition/drug-addiction-treatment-in-united-states/types-treatment-programs

Schmidt, B. (2012). *The critical importance of good data to improving quality. Patient Safety & Quality Healthcare.* https://www.psqh.com/analysis/the-critical-importance-of-good-data-to-improving-quality/July /August 2012

<<<< >>>>

Test Your Knowledge On Quality and Outcomes Evaluations and Measurements

1. All of the following are components of a quality improvement program except:

    A. Systematic

    B. Data-driven

    C. Objective

    D. Fault finding efforts

2. Which survey is given to understand the patients' perspective of their hospital experience?

    A. Agency for Healthcare Research and Quality Mimi Survey (AHRQ)

    B. SurveyMonkey Hospital Perspective

    C. Hospital Consumer Assessment of Healthcare Providers and Systems (HCAHPS)

    D. CMS Centers for Medicare and Medicaid

3. Indicators provide all of the following except:

    A. A quantitative starting point for clinicians

    B. A definitive answer to errors for Quality Management Teams

    C. Suggest good quality care or identify potential problems

    D. Objective measurement

4. Monitoring healthcare quality is impossible without the use of:

    A. Quality Indicators

    B. Incident Reports

    C. Guidelines

    D. Investigations

5. Which quality improvement approach improves quality by reducing waste to increase value?

A. Plan-Do-Study-Act Approach

B. Six Sigma Approach

C. Lean Approach

D. Continuous Quality Improvement Approach

6. Accreditation is:

A. A mandatory process

B. Provided by an internal organization

C. Performed by trained peer reviewers

D. Based on local standard

7. Which accreditation body targets organizations that focus on medical rehabilitation, durable medical equipment, aging services, and behavioral health programs?

A. Joint Commission

B. Commission on Accreditation of Rehabilitation Faculties (CARF)

C. National Committee on Quality Assurance

D. National Quality Forum

8. Which quality improvement accreditation organization supports Healthcare Effectiveness Data and Information Set (HEDIS)?

A. URAC

B. Joint Commission

C. Commission on Accreditation of Rehabilitation Facilities (CARF)

D. National Committee for Quality Assurance (NCQA)

9. Quality Indicators can be used to:

   A. Identify variances

   B. Identify errors

   C. Identify best practices

   D. Identify core measures

10. When interpreting data, what two elements must be taken into consideration?

    A. Consistency and intent

    B. Validity and reliability

    C. Repletion and rationale

    D. Intent and validity

11. The value of Case Management Services are demonstrated in Patient Care Reports as demonstrated in each of the following statements except:

    A. Recording the patient's condition prior to case management involvement and after the case manager's services are delivered to demonstrate a progression of care

    B. Achievement of the case manager's stated goals that were developed with patient input

    C. The patient's condition is relative to the stated goals.

    D. Physician's interventions

12. A Cost-Benefit Analysis:

    A. Formally documents monetary savings related to case management involvement

B. Documents the provider agreement by the managed care organization

C. Explains the cost of care according to the type of insurance the patient has

D. Is the amount of money that can be claimed by the provider after taxes are taken out

13. Which of the following is an example of a hard saving that a case manager can claim?

A. Decreased length of stay after the case manager recommends to the treating physician that the patient is stable and can be transferred to a lower level of care

B. Avoidance of hospital readmission

C. Prevention of medical complications

D. Avoidance of Emergency Department visits

Answer Key

1. Answer: D

Rationale: Quality improvement is not intended to attribute blame, but rather to discover where errors are occurring and to develop systems to prevent errors.

Refer to: Subdomain–Quality and Performance Improvement Concepts.

2. Answer: C

Rationale: Hospital Consumer Assessment of Healthcare Providers and Systems (HCAHPS) is a nationally known standardized survey of patients' perspectives of their hospital experience.

Refer to: Subdomain–Data Interpretation and Reporting.

3. Answer: B

Rationale: Indicators themselves do not provide definitive answers but they do suggest good quality care or potential problems.

Refer to: Subdomain–Quality Indicators and Applications.

4. Answer: A

Rationale: Monitoring health care quality is impossible without quality indicators.

Refer to: Subdomain–Quality Indicators and Applications.

5. Answer: C

Rationale: The Lean approach to quality improvement emphasizes reducing waste to increase value.

Refer to: Subdomain: Quality Indicators and Applications

6. Answer: C

Rationale: Accreditation is usually a voluntary process, provided by an external organization by trained peer reviewers to evaluate a healthcare organization's compliance with nationally accepted standards.

Refer to: Subdomain–Accreditation Standards and Requirements.

7. Answer: B

Rationale: The Commission on Accreditation of Rehabilitation Facilities (CARF) is an independent, non-profit accreditor of health and human services. CARF provides accreditation in the following services: medical rehabilitation, durable medical equipment, aging services, and behavioral health programs.

Refer to: Subdomain–Sources of Quality Indicators.

8. Answer: D

Rationale: The National Committee for Quality Assurance (NCQA) supports and maintains a collection of standardized performance measures known as Health Plan Employer Data and Information Set or HEDIS.

Refer to: Subdomain–Data Interpretation and Reporting.

9. Answer: A

Rationale: The Quality Indicators established and maintained by the Agency for Healthcare Research and Quality are evidence-based and can be used to identify variances in the quality of care on both an inpatient and outpatient basis.

Refer to: Subdomain–Sources of Quality Indicators.

10. Answer B.

Rationale: When interpreting data, validity, and reliability must be taken into consideration.

Refer to: Subdomain–Data Interpretation and Reporting.

11. Answer: D

Rationale: Patient Reports are important as this is where case managers document the value of case management involvement. All of the following choices are correct except the statement "Physician intervention," as this statement does not take into account the case manager's role in the case. To claim an outcome, the case manager must show involvement.

Refer to: Subdomain–Data Interpretation and Reporting.

12. Answer: A

Rationale: A cost-benefit analysis formally documents monetary savings related to case management involvement. They can be hard or soft savings.

Refer to: Subdomain–Cost-Benefit Analysis.

13. Answer: A

Rationale: A is the only answer that provides an example of hard saving that a case manager can claim. The others are examples of soft savings.

Refer to: Subdomain–Cost-Benefit Analysis.

Chapter Six:
Rehabilitation Concepts and Strategies

Rehabilitation Concepts and Strategies comprise 11% of the exam with between 14 and 18 questions on this topic.

****

Case managers need to have a basic understanding of the various rehabilitation options available for medical, vocational, and substance use rehabilitation as well as who is best served by each. In addition, they also need to be familiar with the different levels of care available for each type of rehabilitation.

>>>> <<<<

Rehabilitation Concepts

Substance Use Rehabilitation

According to the National Institute on Drug Abuse (NIDA, 2018), the first stage in the treatment of substance use is usually detoxification and medical management of withdrawal. It is designed to manage the acute and potentially dangerous physiological effects of stopping drug use. Detoxification is often managed with medications administered by a physician in an inpatient or outpatient setting.

Detoxification alone does not address the psychological, social, and behavioral problems associated with addiction and therefore does not typically produce lasting behavioral change necessary for recovery. Therefore it should be followed by ongoing drug addiction treatment. This can be in the form of:

- Long-term residential treatment, usually lasting 6-12 months
- Short-term residential treatment
- Outpatient treatment programs
- Group counseling
- Individual counseling

Community-based programs such as Alcoholics Anonymous and Narcotics Anonymous have been found to be the most successful in treating substance abuse. Inpatient hospitalization for substance abuse is not usually the preferred method of treatment (NIDA, 2018).

Vocational Rehabilitation

Vocational rehabilitation is a process that aims to return workers with some type of disability to work. It enables people with functional, psychological, developmental, cognitive, and/or emotional limitations or health disabilities to overcome the limitation(s) and return to employment in a prior or new job.

Return To Work Strategies

After a work-related injury, the goal is for the worker to achieve maximum medical improvement and to return to work as soon as possible. The return to work options are evaluated in the following order:

1. Same job, same employer

2. Modified job, same employer

3. Different job, same employer, using transferable skills

4. Same job, different employer

5. Different job, different employer, using transferable skills

6. Training for different job with same or different employer

7. Self-employment

Work Hardening and Work Conditioning

An employee who has recovered from his injury may need work conditioning or work hardening to be able to return to pre-injury duties. These therapies are ideal for patients that have already progressed through traditional physical therapy but still lack full function in relation to the specific job required duties.

Work hardening is an individualized, highly structured program designed to help workers return to their pre-injury work in a safe and timely manner. It focuses on work endurance by progressively increasing tolerance with conditioning exercises including; strengthening and flexibility exercises, cardiovascular conditioning, spine and joint stabilization exercises, and job task training such as pushing, pulling, bending, twisting, or lifting. A job analysis or on-site observation of the worker's job may be performed to identify goals related to job functions. Work hardening is multidisciplinary and can include physical therapists, occupational therapists, psychologists, and vocational specialists.

Work conditioning is designed to restore systemic neurological, cardiopulmonary, and musculoskeletal functions to enable the injured worker to return to work. This includes strength, mobility, range of motion, endurance, motor control, power, and aerobic capacity/endurance. It is done under the direction of a physical therapist in a therapy setting. Work conditioning differs from work hardening in that the focus is not on specific tasks the client must perform (for example, lifting a 20-pound box and placing it on a shelf), but rather on building the strength required to lift anything.

If the client has reached Medical Maximum Improvement (MMI) and cannot perform the essential duties of the job, with or without accommodation, a Transferable Skills Analysis can be completed to document current and projected employment based on the skills, abilities, and aptitude of the client.

Rehabilitation After Hospitalization or an Acute Health Condition

Following a prolonged hospitalization or an acute illness or injury, such as a stroke or hip fracture, patients are at risk of experiencing a significant loss of functioning. This risk is increased in critically ill patients, patients with complications or long-term intensive care stays, patients with disabilities or preexisting chronic conditions, and the elderly. Early identification of rehabilitation needs and proactive rehabilitation can reduce healthcare costs. Rehabilitation can occur at the acute-level hospital, the non-acute inpatient setting, or in the community.

**See Vocational and Rehabilitation Service Delivery Systems for more information on care settings

Assessment of Physical Functioning

The functional assessment is an important part of rehabilitation. It guides the treatment types and duration, measures outcomes, estimates the amount of care to be provided by others, and provides documentation for payment for care. The Functional Independence Measures instrument (FIM) assesses adult inpatients, while the WeeFIM is used for children.

Functional Independence Measures Instrument (FIM)

FIM is an 18 item instrument used in the inpatient rehab setting and measures the individual's level of independence/dependence in the areas of:

- Self-care (e.g., eating, grooming, bathing, upper body dressing, lower body dressing)
- Toileting (e.g., bladder control, sphincter control)
- Transfers (e.g., bed/chair/wheelchair, toilet, tub/shower)
- Locomotion (e.g., walk, wheelchair, stairs)
- Communication (e.g., comprehension, expression)
- Social cognition (e.g., social interaction, problem-solving, memory)

Clinicians score patients from 1-7, with 7 indicating complete independence and 1 indicating total assist from another person. The instrument allows healthcare professionals to evaluate the amount of assistance required by a client to safely and effectively perform basic life functions.

It is completed within 72 hours of admission to rehabilitation, at regular intervals during rehabilitation, and within 72 hours of discharge. This gages the effectiveness of the treatment plan as the client should show improvement. Clinicians who typically complete the FIM and assign scores include physical therapists, occupational therapists, nurses, psychologists, and social workers.

The instrument is copyrighted and maintained by the Uniform Data System for Medical Rehabilitation (UDSMR), which is a division of the University of Buffalo Foundation Activities, Inc.

WeeFIM

The WeeFIM assesses children in the same areas as the FIM and uses the same rating scale. It is used for children without disabilities ages 6 months to 7 years, and in children with developmental disabilities ages 6 months to 12 years.

Vocational and Rehabilitation Service Delivery Systems

Medical Rehabilitation

Medical inpatient rehabilitation may be provided in a medical hospital, a long-term acute care hospital, a freestanding inpatient rehabilitation hospital, or a skilled nursing facility. The setting is determined by the client's medical and functional status and the level of care the facility can provide.

The medical hospital level is for patients with an acute medical need that requires ongoing medical care. Rehabilitation such as physical therapy, occupational therapy, speech therapy, and cognitive rehabilitation are provided, but medical care is the priority. This level of care can be delivered in two hospital settings: acute care hospital or long-term acute care hospital.

The inpatient rehabilitation hospital provides intense, multidisciplinary therapy to patients with a functional loss due to factors such as injury, illness, or deconditioning. The primary focus is to restore the client to self-sufficiency or maximum possible functional independence. These hospitals utilize an interdisciplinary team to provide intensive rehabilitation in the areas of physical therapy, occupational therapy, speech therapy, cognitive therapy, respiratory therapy, psychology services, and/or prosthetic/orthotic services. To qualify for this level of care, patients must be able to tolerate a minimum of three hours of therapy per day, five to seven days per week, and be medically stable.

Skilled nursing facilities (SNF) provide rehabilitation services such as physical therapy, occupational therapy, and speech therapy, at a less intense level than inpatient rehabilitation hospitals. Patients who need rehabilitation after injury or hospitalization but cannot tolerate three hours of therapy per day may benefit from the SNF level of rehabilitation. Patients must be medically stable to qualify for SNF care.

Community Medical Rehabilitation

Patients who do not require the inpatient level of care can still benefit from rehabilitation services utilizing outpatient rehabilitation or home health services.

Day program – An outpatient program for patients who no longer require hospitalization but still need intensive, coordinated rehabilitation for several hours per day.

Outpatient rehabilitation – Patients travel to a clinic or hospital to attend sessions and return home the same day. Typically, a therapy session lasts from 30 minutes to an hour.

Home health – Therapy is provided in the patient's home for up to one hour per discipline per visit. Visits are usually made up to three times per week. To qualify for home health care, the patient must be homebound, meaning taxing effort is required to leave the home. A person may leave home for medical treatment or short, infrequent non-medical reasons, such as attending religious services.

Vocational Rehabilitation

Vocational rehabilitation uses counselors and professionals/specialists to aid the client in securing meaningful employment. Vocational rehabilitation counselors specialize in vocational counseling and provide group and individual counseling, create job plans, and guide clients to help them achieve their employment goals. Vocational rehabilitation professionals, also known as Vocational Rehabilitation Specialists (VRS), are professionals who work with an interdisciplinary healthcare team to help eligible clients with disabilities attain and maintain competitive employment; and overcome psychological, developmental, cognitive, and health barriers so that these individuals are able to obtain meaningful jobs and increase their independence.

Federal-state governments also have eligibility-based, career development programs. These provide a wide range of individualized services to eligible individuals with disabilities. The individuals acquire skills, attitudes, and resources needed to obtain and keep a job.

To be eligible for federal-state vocational rehabilitation services, federal regulations require the individual to be disabled and able to benefit from vocational rehabilitation services. The disability must be a physical or mental impairment that is a substantial barrier to employment. Those receiving Supplemental Security Income (SSI) and/or Social Security Disability Insurance (SSDI) are presumed eligible unless their disabilities are too severe for them to benefit from vocational rehabilitation (defined as being unable to achieve employment).

The Ticket to Work Program exists for clients aged 18 to 64 who want to return to work, but currently receive Social Security benefits based on disability under the Social Security Disability Insurance (SSDI) program and/or the Supplemental Security Income (SSI) program. It is a voluntary program that provides expanded options for accessing employment services, vocational rehabilitation services, or other support services needed to enter, maintain, and advance in employment.

These services include training, career counseling, vocational rehabilitation, job placement, and ongoing support services necessary to achieve a work goal. The ultimate goal of the program is to eliminate the need for Social Security disability cash benefits while allowing the client to maintain his or her Medicare or Medicaid benefits.

***More information can be found at https://yourtickettowork.ssa.gov/index.html

Supported Employment

Supported employment is paid, competitive employment in an integrated setting with ongoing support for individuals with the most severe disabilities (e.g., psychiatric or intellectual disability, significant learning disabilities, traumatic brain injury, deafness and blindness, extreme mobility impairments, and other severe disabilities). Because of the nature and severity of these disabilities, workers need on-going support services in order to obtain, perform, and retain their jobs. Supported employment provides assistance such as job coaching, job placement, specialized job training, on-site assistive technology, transportation, help interacting with employers, and individually tailored supervision.

Supported employment provides a vehicle for eligible individuals to enter competitive employment, where they would otherwise be unable to do so due to the impact of their disabling conditions.

Work Adjustment

The focus of work adjustment is on attitude, behavior, and social skills for clients with behavioral health issues. Work adjustment can be done individually or in a group setting. Real or simulated work activity is performed under close supervision at a rehabilitation facility or work setting. The goal is to improve problems that prevent the client from obtaining employment, such as attendance, punctuality, hygiene, or interpersonal relationship skills. Work adjustment might be used after a traumatic brain injury, for example, wherein the worker has developed behavioral issues.

Vocational Aspects of Disability(ies) and Illnesses

The vocational aspects of a chronic illness or disability can be a challenge to manage. Along with medical and psychological issues, the reduction or loss of income can place a huge burden on the client and his family. Clients usually exhaust any paid time off first. If the client is expected to be out of work for an extended period of time, he will want to apply for protection under the Family and Medical Leave Act (FMLA). FMLA is not a source of income, but it does protect the employee's job.

Workers' compensation clients have an advantage over clients who suffer from an illness: They are afforded benefits to get them through. Persons who are injured outside of work or suffer a prolonged illness can lose their medical and other benefits, as well as their income, if they cannot return to work or be approved for disability.

According to the U.S. Department of Health and Human Services, the employment rate for adults with disabilities is significantly lower than for those without disabilities. The most frequently reported reasons for difficulty in obtaining employment are lack of available, appropriate jobs, followed by lack of transportation. Many individuals need some accommodation, such as accessible parking or transportation, elevators, or specially designed workstations.

Job Analysis

A functional job analysis is the process of collecting data to define a person's job requirements and essential and nonessential job duties. This data can be collected from interviews with workers and supervisors, on-site observations, and analysis of company job descriptions. It provides detailed information related to major tasks, as well as the physical, cognitive, and behavioral capacities required to perform the job. Items examined in the job analysis may include: essential duties of the job, tools and equipment used, and amount of time spent standing, walking, sitting, operating a vehicle, climbing, reaching, bending, kneeling, and lifting. Along with specific tasks, the job analysis also includes details regarding scheduling, location, equipment needed, and required competencies.

In rehabilitation, the goal of the job analysis is to identify essential job functions and requirements to satisfactorily perform the work. Job requirements must be the focus, not the individual worker's skills. Once the job analysis has identified the required skills, competencies, and qualifications of the job, a plan can be created to provide training or work accommodations to get the injured worker back to work.

Essential job functions are the basic duties fundamental to the job, and the employee must be able to perform them with or without reasonable accommodations. The most obvious functions are those the position exists to perform. For example, an obvious job function for a cashier is to exchange money with customers. Other information provided in the job analysis include a reference to the written job description, the amount of time spent performing the function(s), and the consequences if this employee is not required to perform a particular function.

The job analysis may be performed by one discipline or an interdisciplinary rehabilitation team. Disciplines that often perform a rehabilitation job analysis include:

- Physical therapists
- Occupational therapists
- Vocational rehabilitation specialists
- Ergonomists

Job Modification/Job Accommodation

The terms job modification and job accommodation are often used interchangeably. To differentiate, however, a job modification is an across the board change to the job description, targeting skills. Examples include restructuring the job, eliminating marginal job functions, sharing job duties, or modifying company policy. Job accommodations are more individualized and focus on access. Examples include voice recognition software or an adjustable height desk to accommodate a wheelchair. Because most of the literature, as well as most case managers, use either accommodation or modification to mean both, the term accommodation will be used for the remainder of this section.

Job Accommodation Process:

1. Request accommodation: The person with the disability is responsible for requesting the accommodation.

2. Identify functional limitations: Determine where the functional limitations intersect with the job duties; that is, which tasks the person cannot perform without accommodation.

3. Identify accommodations: Discuss options with the employee. Often the accommodation is obvious or something the employee has used before successfully, but creative collaboration, extensive investigation, or outside assistance may be needed.

4. Determine reasonable solutions: The ADA requires employers to provide reasonable accommodations for qualified applicants or employees with disabilities, unless doing so would cause undue hardship for the employer. Undue hardship can refer to accommodations that cause financial difficulty, are disruptive to the workplace, or fundamentally change the operation of the business.

5. Make accommodation: The employee's preferences should be taken into account, but ultimately the employer will determine which accommodation is put into effect based on cost, business feasibility, and effectiveness.

6. Monitor effectiveness: If the desired outcome is not achieved, the employee and the employer should start the process again.

The Job Accommodations Network (JAN) is a consulting service provided by the U.S. Department of Labor's Office of Disability Employment Policy (ODEP) that provides free information on job accommodations. JAN's website states, "Working toward practical solutions that benefit both employer and employee, JAN helps people with disabilities enhance their employability, and shows employers how to capitalize on the value and talent that people with disabilities add to the workplace" (JAN, 2020). JAN has an online resource, the Searchable Online Accommodation Resource (SOAR) which is designed to let users explore various accommodation options. This tool can be found at https://askjan.org/soar.cfm

Data collected on the cost of accommodations show that more than half of all accommodations cost nothing. For modifications that do have a cost, the majority are under $500, and tax incentives and funding are available through several organizations to help offset the expense.

Accommodations are not limited to adjustment or modifications of physical equipment. The Americans with Disabilities Act lists these six categories of accommodations:

- Job restructuring – Adjustments to work procedures
- Assistive devices – Equipment that helps the employee complete the task
- Training – Helps an employee learn or relearn job duties
- Personal assistant – A person who helps an employee with job duties
- Building modification – Alterations to the physical environment that allow equal access to the facility
- Job reassignment – Temporary or permanent transfer of task assignment, or sharing jobs with other employees

Transitional Work Duty

After a work injury, an employee may need some assistance before he is able to return to the job duties he had prior to the injury. If he is able to work but at a lower capacity than before the injury, the worker may be a candidate for Transitional Work Duty (TWD). This would be appropriate for a police officer who broke his leg, for example. He is able to work, but not in his normal job function. He could be placed in a desk job until he is able to return to his normal job duties.

TWD allows an injured employee to return to productive work with their employer while under the care of rehabilitation professionals. The employer creates a value-added temporary position based on the knowledge and skills of the employee. The work must conform to the restrictions put in place by the employee's treating physician. Only employees with temporary injuries who will eventually be able to return to their normal full-time duties are eligible for TWD.

Life Care Planning

If the injury, condition, or disability is complex, catastrophic, or life-altering a life care plan may need to be created. According to the International Association of Rehabilitation Professionals (IARP), "the life care plan is a dynamic document based on published standards of practice, comprehensive assessment, data analysis, and research, which provides an organized, concise plan for current and future needs with associated costs for individuals who have experienced catastrophic injury or have chronic health care needs. (International Conference on Life Care Planning and the International Academy of Life Care Planners. Adopted 1998, April.)" (IARP, 2020).

The ultimate goal of the life care plan is to promote and maintain the client's health, safety, well-being, and quality of life. It applies a consistent methodology for analyzing all of the actual present and potential future needs as well as their associated expenses dictated by the onset of catastrophic disability through to the end of life expectancy.

Functional Capacity Evaluation (FCE)

CCMC in their glossary of terms defines Functional Capacity Evaluation (FCE) as "a systematic process of assessing an individual's physical capacities and functional abilities. The FCE matches human performance levels to the demands of a specific job or work activity or occupation. It establishes the physical level of work an individual can perform" (CCMC, 2017).

The FCE is used to directly measure the patient's physical ability to perform work-related activities. The worker is examined as he completes activities, directly measuring the physical level of work the individual can perform. It is an objective tool that is dependent on the motivation, cognitive awareness, and sincerity of effort of the participant and only reflects what he is able or willing to do at the time of the evaluation. Factors that may influence this include sincerity of effort, motivation, and mental alertness.

The FCE is done in a structured setting, not the place of work, and is performed by an independent physical therapist, occupational therapist, or physician, not the treating clinician.

During the FCE, the patient is evaluated as he performs activities required for his job. This may include, but is not limited to:

- Squatting
- Sitting
- Pushing
- Pulling
- Turning
- Standing
- Kneeling
- Balancing
- Navigating stairs
- Gripping/Grasping

The amount of time the patient requires to perform each of these tasks is important.

The FCE is a comprehensive exam, covering all physical demands required of the employee. Because of this, it can be used as part of the initial assessment as well as to:

- Prepare a work conditioning plan
- Assess progress

- Evaluate the capacity for returning to the current job
- Plan job modification(s) or accommodation(s)
- Manage job placement
- Determine occupational disability status

Adaptive Technologies

Assistive devices include any tool that is designed, made, or adapted to assist a person to perform a particular task. Assistive or adaptive technology is an item, product system, or piece of equipment that is used to increase, maintain, or improve functional capabilities of individuals with disabilities.

The use of the device allows the individual with impaired abilities or functional limitations greater independence in performing activities. They can be high-tech, such as computers and hearing aids, or as simple as a cane or reacher. The purpose of the device is to improve function and independence. They can also be used as job accommodations.

Aids for physical disabilities that affect mobility include:
- Canes
- Crutches
- Walkers
- Scooters
- Manual wheelchairs
- Power wheelchairs

There are several points to consider when helping a client choose a mobility device (that is, a manual wheelchair, power wheelchair, or scooter). It is important to understand the client's insurance coverage for the various devices, such as the criteria for medical necessity and coverage for maintenance and repairs.

Manual wheelchairs are the least expensive and are lightweight, making them much more portable than power chairs. On the other hand, they require sufficient upper-body strength to self-propel, making them unsuitable for some clients.

For clients who are unable to self-propel, a scooter or power wheelchair can be a better option. Power wheelchairs offer the greatest variety of options and accessories to customize the chair to the needs of the client, but they can be much more expensive than manual wheelchairs. They also tend to be very heavy, requiring the use of a power lift for transport. Scooters are often faster but provide less stability than power wheelchairs. Many scooters can disassemble quickly for transport.

Both scooters and power wheelchairs are battery operated and require regular charging and maintenance. Before purchasing a scooter or power chair, the client should be evaluated by a physical therapist to ensure he will be able to use the device.

Computer software and hardware can allow people with sensory or motor impairments to use computers. This includes:

- Alternate keyboard
- Voice recognition programs
- Screen readers
- Screen enlargement applications

Devices to assist with orientation to person, place, and time include:

- Clocks
- Calendars
- Smartphones
- Memory books
- Location devices

A prosthetic device is an artificial substitute or replacement part for a missing or impaired part of the body and includes:

- Hip, knee, or other joint replacement
- Lens replacement following cataract surgery
- Breast implants following mastectomy
- Tooth
- Eye
- Artificial arm or leg

Telecommunication devices for the deaf (TDD) include:

- Teletypewriter (TTY)
- Text Telephone Device (TTD)

The acronyms TDD, TTY, and TTD are used interchangeably to refer to any type of text-based telecommunications equipment used by someone with hearing or speech difficulties. Both the sender and the receiver of the message need the equipment.

There are also relay services to allow a hearing-impaired person with a TDD to communicate with another party who does not have a TDD. The operator at the relay service uses TDD equipment to communicate with the hearing-impaired person and a telephone to communicate with the other party, acting as an interpreter. There are also video relay services that allow the hearing impaired person to communicate in American Sign Language. The popularity of cell phones and texting has made communication for the deaf much easier, as no special equipment is needed.

Other types of assistive devices include:

- Hearing aids
- Page-turners
- Book-holders
- Adapted pencil grips
- Closed captioning
- Reachers

BONUS

I highly recommend that you access the free Companion Workbook that I've created for you. You can access it at

CCMcertificationMadeEasy.com

The free Companion Workbook follows along with the book and replaces key words and phrases with blank lines. Writing these words and phrases into the blank lines helps you to remember them.

References

Commission for Case Management Certification. (2017). *Glossary of terms.* https://ccmcertification.org/get-certified/exam-study-materials/ccmc-glossary

International Association of Rehabilitation Professionals. (n.d.). *Life Care Planning FAQ.* Retrieved June 20, 2020, from https://connect.rehabpro.org/lcp/about/new-item/new-item

U.S. Department of Labor. (n.d.). Job Accommodation Network. https://askjan.org/

Test Your Knowledge On Rehabilitation Concepts and Strategies

1. The purpose of assistive technologies is to:

   A. Improve function and independence

   B. Ensure a safe environment

   C. Prevent complications of immobility

   D. Improve the patient's morale

2. Prosthetic devices include all of the following except:

   A. Tooth

   B. Eye

   C. Artificial leg or arm

   D. Kidney

3. Early identification of rehabilitation needs and proactive rehabilitation can:

   A. Ensure an early discharge

   B. Allow the patient to avoid a disability

   C. Reduce healthcare costs

   D. Prevent depression

4. Which of the following is true regarding the functional assessment in regards to rehabilitation?

   A. It can be used to guide the treatment and measure outcomes

   B. It predicts disability

   C. Aids the caregiver to decide if the patient needs a nursing home

   D. Provides documentation that will allow the patient to be placed on Social Security Disability

5. The Wee-FIM assesses:

   A. Adults

   B. Seniors

   C. Children

   D. All age Groups

6. Case managers use what criteria to make a recommendation on the type of rehabilitation program the patient should go to?

   A. The type of insurance the patient has

   B. The patient's medical and functional status and the level of care the facility can provide

   C. The cost of the facility

   D. The case manager follows the orders of the treating physician

7. Supported employment is:

   A. Paid, competitive employment in an integrated setting with ongoing support for individuals with severe disabilities

   B. Paid, competitive employment in a traditional setting for individuals with severe disabilities

   C. Paid, competitive employment in an integrated setting with ongoing support for individuals leaving drug rehab

   D. Non-paid employment for people with severe disabilities

8. In the event of a work-related injury, the goal of the case manager is to:

   A. Provide emergency care to limit the extent of the injury

   B. Return the patient to work as quickly as possible

C. Give the patient time off until they recover

D. Have the patient seen by a medical doctor to avoid a lawsuit

9. If a client has reached Maximum Medical Improvement, and cannot perform the essential duties of their job, with or without accommodations, what is the next step?

A. The claims adjuster will settle the case.

B. A transferable skills analysis can be completed to document current and projected employment based on the skills, abilities, and aptitude of the client

C. An application for Social Security should be started.

D. The case manager should close the case as nothing else can be done

10. What type of work can be offered to an injured worker who is not ready to return to their main job?

A. Sheltered Employment

B. Transitional Work Duty

C. Supported Work Duty

D. Per-Diem work

11. Work Adjustment focuses on all of the following except:

A. Attitude

B. Behavior

C. Endurance

D. Social skills

12. The point at which the health or medical condition of a worker who has sustained a work-related injury or illness has stabilized, and further improvements are considered unlikely despite continued care and treatment is:

    A. Maximum Medical Improvement

    B. Maximum Medical Stability

    C. Complete Medical Improvement

    D. Medical Improvement Stability

13. Which would be most appropriate for a 52-year-old nurse who has a broken leg as the result of a work-related injury?

    A. Work hardening

    B. Work adjustment

    C. Transitional Work Duty

    D. Temporary Total Disability

14. The goal of the job analysis in work rehabilitation is to identify:

    A. Essential job functions and requirements

    B. The strengths and abilities of the employee

    C. The company culture

    D. Average productivity per employee

Answer Key

1. Answer: A

   Rationale: Assistive technology is an item, product system, or piece of equipment that is used to increase, maintain, or improve functional capabilities of individuals with disabilities. All of the others may be true, but A explains the purpose.

   Refer to: CCMC Glossary of Terms.

2. Answer D

   Rationale: A prosthetic device is an artificial substitute or replacement part for a missing or impaired part of the body, such as a tooth, eye, or artificial leg or arm.

   Refer to: Subdomain–Adaptive Technologies.

3. Answer: C

   Rationale: Early identification and getting a patient into a rehabilitation facility can reduce costs. The others may be true, but C is the best answer.

   Refer to: Subdomain–Rehabilitation After Hospitalization or an Acute Health Condition.

4. Answer: A

   Rationale: The functional assessment is an important part of rehabilitation. It guides the treatment types and duration, measures outcomes, estimates the amount of care to be provided by others, and provides documentation for payment for care.

   Refer to: Subdomain–Rehabilitation After Hospitalization or an Acute Health Condition.

5. Answer: C

   Rationale: The WeeFIM tool assesses children in the same areas as the FIM that is used in adult medicine and uses the same rating scale.

Refer to: Subdomain–Rehabilitation After Hospitalization or an Acute Health Condition.

6. Answer: B

Rationale: A professional Case Manager collaborates with the treatment team to understand the patient's medical and functional status when deciding on which type of rehabilitation program the patient should go.

Refer to: Subdomain–Vocational and Rehabilitation Service Delivery Systems.

7. Answer: A

Rationale: Supported employment is a paid, competitive employment program in an integrated setting with ongoing support for individuals with the most severe disabilities.

Refer to: Subdomain–Vocational and Rehabilitation Service Delivery Systems.

8. Answer: B

Rationale: In the event of a work-related injury, the goal of the case manager is to return the injured worker to work as quickly as possible.

Refer to: Subdomain–Rehabilitation Concepts and Strategies.

9. Answer: B

Rationale: A transferable skills analysis can give the case manager, the vocational specialist, the claims adjustor, and the treatment team additional information that may help with return to work options.

Refer to: Subdomain–Rehabilitation Concepts and Strategies.

10. Answer B

Rationale: Transitional Work Duty allows someone who is able to work, but not at their regular job due to their work-related injury, to return to work. This is a temporary solution that allows the injured worker to return to work while healing from their injury.

Refer to: Subdomain–Vocational Aspects of Disability(ies) and Illnesses.

11. Answer: C

Rationale: The focus of work adjustment is on attitude, behavioral, and social skills for clients with behavioral health issues.

Refer to: Subdomain–Vocational and Rehabilitation Service Delivery Systems.

12. Answer: A

Rationale: Maximum Medical Improvement is defined as the point at which the health or medical condition of a worker who has sustained a work-related injury or illness has stabilized and further improvements are considered unlikely despite continued care and treatment. The treating physician at this time usually explains that no other reasonable treatment can be done to help the worker improve.

Refer to: CCMC Glossary of Terms.

13. Answer: C

Rationale: Transitional work duty (TWD) allows an injured employee to return to work. The employer will create a temporary position that conforms to the restrictions put in place by the employee's treating physician.

Refer to: Subdomain–Vocational Aspects of Disability(ies) and Illnesses.

14. Answer: A

Rationale: The primary focus of a job analysis is identifying the essential functions and requirements of the job. This may include essential duties, tasks, skills, tools and equipment used, environment, and scheduling.

Refer to: CCMC Glossary of Terms.

Chapter Seven:
Ethical, Legal, and Practice Standards

Ethical, Legal, and Practice Standards comprise 17% of the exam with between 23 and 27 questions on this topic.

****

Case managers are licensed professionals who are obligated to work within ethical, legal, and practice standards as required by their license, governing bodies, and accrediting organizations. The board-certified case manager must have a good understanding of these standards; therefore, the Commission for Case Management Certification (CCMC) dedicates 17% of the CCM Exam to this topic.

Because of the board-certified case manager's role in protecting the rights, dignity, and public interest of her clients, the CCMC now requires CCMs to earn ethics-related continuing education credits for recertification.

Ethics Related to Care Delivery

Principles

There are five basic ethical principles; beneficence, nonmaleficence, autonomy, justice, and fidelity. Beneficence, to do good, is a core principle of client advocacy in that it involves taking positive action to help others. Nonmaleficence, to do no harm, is demonstrated by working toward quality care outcomes.

Autonomy is the ethical principle that respects the individual's rights to make their own decisions and to self-determine a course of action. Justice is to treat others fairly and equally, and also extends to the equitable access to resources and treatment. And fidelity is to follow-through, keeping commitments and promises.

Advocacy

The role of the case manager as a client advocate stems from the principle of client autonomy. The needs of the client, as the client sees them, are primary. The case manager collaborates with the autonomous client with the goal of fostering and encouraging the client's independence and self-determination. This involves informing the client of his options and supporting his decisions. Once the client has made an informed decision, the case manager advocates for the client by speaking on their behalf to make sure their decisions are understood and supported.

Experimental Treatment

Experimental treatments come with great potential for ethical issues. An ethical review committee should evaluate experimental treatments before they are offered to a patient. The committee will determine if the anticipated social value justifies possible harm. Any patient receiving experimental treatment must give informed consent after all aspects of care, including the likelihood of harm and the severity of the harm, are disclosed. There must also be an equitable system to select patients to participate in the experimental treatment.

End of Life

With the advances of medical intervention, end of life care is rife with potential ethical dilemmas, ranging from the use of heroic measures to sustain life to assisted suicide. Other ethical issues at the end of life can be related to advance directives, pain control, prolonging life, avoiding prolonged suffering, artificial nutrition and hydration, and forgoing treatment.

Case managers can help clients and families make informed decisions regarding end of life care that can prevent or relieve suffering and make an impact on the costs that are often associated with end of life care. The case manager should understand the client's wishes regarding end of life care. Once these wishes are understood, the case manager can provide education as to the options available and how to ensure the client's wishes are acted on. This could be in the form of a palliative care consult, hospice, and/or advance directives such as a Durable Power of Attorney, Living Will, and/or Do Not Resuscitate.

Advance Directives

An advance directive is a legally executed document that explains the client's healthcare-related wishes. It is created while the client is competent and is used if the client is unable to make decisions due to incapacity or incompetence.

Advance directives come in two forms, those that dictate what kind of medical treatment to be given or withheld such as a living will or do not resuscitate, and those that appoint an agent or proxy to make healthcare decisions. Both forms only go into effect if the person is unable to make the decision for themselves. Every state has its own advance directive forms and requirements. Next is a description of the different types of advance directives available. It is important to note that the names may vary slightly between states and organizations.

Living Will

A living will states which specific life-sustaining medical treatments the designated person would like to receive or have withheld if death from a terminal condition is imminent, or if the client is in a permanent vegetative state. These treatments can include, but are not limited to:

- Mechanical ventilation
- Dialysis
- Tube feedings
- IV fluids
- Antibiotics
- CPR

Healthcare Power of Attorney/Medical Durable Power of Attorney

This type of advance directive designates who is to make healthcare decisions on behalf of the person if they are unable to make decisions for themselves.

Do Not Resuscitate/Do Not Attempt Resuscitation/Allow Natural Death

A do not resuscitate (DNR), do not attempt resuscitation (DNAR), or allow natural death (AND) is another type of advance directive that is a request not to have CPR attempted.

Patient Self-Determination Act

The Patient Self-Determination Act (PSDA) amends titles XVIII (Medicare) and XIX (Medicaid) of the Social Security Act. It requires all hospitals, skilled nursing facilities, home health agencies, hospice programs, and health maintenance organizations that receive Medicare and Medicaid reimbursement to recognize the living will and durable power of attorney for healthcare. Under the PSDA they must:

- Ask patients if they have an advance directive
- Inform the patient of their rights under state law to make decisions concerning their medical care
- Not discriminate against persons who have executed an advance directive
- Ensure legally valid advance directives are implemented to the extent permitted by state law
- Provide educational programs for staff, patients, and the community on ethical issues concerning patient self-determination and advance directives

**Also see the section on Hospice, Palliative, and End of Life Care in the chapter Care Delivery and Reimbursement Methods.

Refusal of Treatment

Clients may refuse treatment and have the legal right to do so. The Patient's Bill of Rights is a law that ensures all clients have the right to agree to or refuse treatment and be informed of the consequences of such decisions.

Ethics Related to Professional Practice

Cultural and Linguistic Sensitivity

CMSA in their Standards of Practice for Case Management (Revised 2016) address cultural and linguistic sensitivity in their Standard on Cultural Competence. It states that the professional case manager should maintain awareness of and be responsive to the cultural and linguistic diversity of the demographics of her work setting and to the specific client and/or caregiver needs.

How Demonstrated:

- Evidence of communicating in an effective, respectful, and sensitive manner, and in accordance with the client's cultural and linguistic context.

- Assessments, goal-setting, and development of a case management plan of care to accommodate each client's cultural and linguistic needs and preference of services.

- Identified appropriate resources to enhance the client's access to care and improve healthcare outcomes. These may include the use of interpreters and health educational materials which apply language and format demonstrative of understanding of the client's cultural and linguistic communication patterns, including but not limited to speech volume, context, tone, kinetics, space, and other similar verbal/non-verbal communication patterns.

- Pursuit of professional education to maintain and advance one's level of cultural competence and effectiveness while working with diverse client populations.

**See Multicultural, Spiritual, and Religious Factors in the chapter Psychosocial Concepts and Support Systems for more on this topic.

Code of Professional Conduct

The Commission for Case Manager Certification Code of Professional Conduct for Case Managers covers five areas:

- The Client Advocate
- Professional Responsibility, comprising competence and conflict of interest, as well as other areas
- Case Manager/Client Relationships, including a description of services, relationships with clients, and termination of services
- Confidentiality, Privacy, Security, and Recordkeeping
- Professional Relationships, including dual relationships, unprofessional behavior, fees, solicitation, and research

The CCMC Code of Professional Conduct for Case Managers is frequently reviewed and revised as necessary. The entire and most recent version can be found on their website: https://ccmcertification.org/about-ccmc/code-

<u>professional-conduct</u>. For your convenience we also have a direct link available at CCMcertificationMadeEasy.com. Below is a general overview.

Board-certified case managers are to serve as client advocates, perform comprehensive assessments to identify needs, and offer options when appropriate. They have a professional responsibility to practice within the boundaries of their role and competence and to participate in ongoing professional development. Any conflict of interest must be fully disclosed to all affected parties, and if any objection is made, the board-certified case manager will withdraw from further participation in the case.

Board-certified case managers are to maintain objectivity in their professional relationships and not impose their values on their clients. Prior to the termination of case management services, board-certified case managers will document notification of discontinuation to all relevant parties. They must also be knowledgeable about and act in accordance with all laws related to their scope of practice. Confidentiality must be maintained regarding the client's protected health information, including storage and disposal of records.

Any dual relationship that exists between the board-certified case manager and the client, payer, employer, friend, relative, research study, and/or other entities must be disclosed. Board-certified case managers may not participate in unprofessional behavior, such as failing to maintain appropriate professional boundaries with the client, disclosing information about a client via social media, committing a crime, and/or engaging in fraud, deceit, or discrimination.

Veracity

CCMC in their Glossary of Terms (2019) defines veracity as a "legal principle that states that a healthcare professional should be honest and give full disclosure; abstain from misrepresentation or deceit; report known lapses of the standards of care to the proper agencies. (Mosby's Dental Dictionary, 2nd Ed, 2008)."

Information used with permission from the Commission for Case Manager Certification®. All rights reserved.

Additional Ethical Considerations for Case Managers

The Case Management Society of America in its 2016 Standards of Practice addresses the standard of Ethics. According to the Standards of Practice, case managers are to behave and practice ethically, adhering to the tenets of the code of ethics that underlies their professional credentials (e.g., nursing, social work, rehabilitation counseling, etc.). Case management ethics are demonstrated by recognizing that:

- A primary obligation is to the clients cared for.
- A secondary obligation is engagement in and maintenance of respectful relationships with coworkers, employers, and other professionals.
- Laws, rules, policies, insurance benefits, and regulations are sometimes in conflict with ethical principles; in such situations, the professional case manager is bound to address the conflicts to the best of her abilities and/ or seek appropriate consultation.

Ethical dilemmas occur when there is no "right" answer. For example, when upholding a law conflicts with a practice standard. Many circumstances can cause ethical issues for case managers, including, but not limited to:

- Client advocacy vs. cost saving
- Case manager's influence on the client
- Client's values conflicting with the case manager's values
- Client autonomy vs. client safety
- Client advocacy vs. family/caregiver wishes
- Advance directives
- Surrogate decision-making
- Refusal of treatment
- Dual relationship - A dual relationship exists when the case manager has responsibilities toward a third party other than the client. (e.g., client/employer, client/provider, client/payer)

To be an ethical dilemma, three conditions must be present.

- There is a decision the individual must make.
- There must be different courses of action to choose from.
- No matter which course of action is taken, an ethical principle is compromised.

Understanding the underlying values and principles of case management is important in resolving ethical dilemmas, whether they are related to end of life issues, experimental treatments, refusal of care, or any other reason. Case management values are based on the belief that it is a means for improving client health, wellness, and autonomy through advocacy, communication, education, identification of service resources, and service facilitation.

The underlying principles of case management are:

- Placing public interest above one's own at all times
- Respecting the rights and inherent dignity of all clients
- Maintaining objectivity in relationships with clients
- Acting with integrity in dealing with other professionals to facilitate maximum benefit for the client
- Maintaining a level of competency that ensures each client will receive appropriate and consistent services for the client's conditions and circumstances
- Obeying laws and regulations

Standards of Practice

The case manager is held to the standards related to their license (social worker or registered nurse, for example) as well as the Case Management Society of America's Standards of Practice for Case Management.

Case Management Society of America Standards of Practice for Case Management (CMSA's SoP)

CMSA's Standards of Practice are the professional standards every professional case manager is held to. For this reason, it is essential that the case manager knows, understands, and practices within these standards. They cover the definition of case management, the philosophy and guiding principles of case management, case management practice settings, components of the case management process, as well as standards of case management.

CMSA's SoP can be downloaded from their website. For your convenience, CMSA has graciously permitted us to add their Standards of Practice for Case Management in the Appendix of this book.

National Association of Social Workers Standards for Case Management

In addition to CMSA's SoP, social worker case managers are also held to the standards created by the National Association of Social Workers (NASW). These standards create clear guidelines, goals, and objectives related to case management in social work practice, research, policy, and education.

The standards cover definitions and guiding principles, the necessary qualifications of the social work case manager, ethics and values, leadership, interdisciplinary collaboration, professional development, and competence among others.

***You can see the complete standards on the NASW website at https://www.socialworkers.org/LinkClick.aspx?fileticket=acrzqmEfhlo%3D&portalid=0

Case Recording and Documentation

The importance of good documentation cannot be overemphasized. A case manager's documentation assists in clinical management, justifies interventions and expenses, and defends against claims of negligence. When documenting, case managers should maintain professional objectivity and document facts, recording quotations when appropriate. Opinions and biases should not be included in the medical record. The best time to document is during or right after the encounter.

What should be documented depends on the setting in which the case manager works. Examples may include but are not limited to, records of:

- Acceptance or refusal of case management services
- Assessments
- Observations
- Monitoring
- Evaluation findings
- Interventions
- Progress with the current treatment
- Modifications to the case management plan, including rationale for the modifications
- Outcomes
- Discharge planning
- Medical stability of the patient within 24 hours of hospital discharge
- Plan of care, including patient/family agreement of
- Patient/family education
- Evidence of continuation of care after discharge from inpatient setting
- Informed consent
- Pre-certifications for procedures
- Advance directives

Additionally, all communication with the following must be documented:

- Patient
- Family
- Insurer/payer

- Vendors
- Other healthcare providers, both inside and outside the organization

Privacy and Confidentiality

A case manager must follow federal, state, and local laws regarding client privacy and confidentiality, as well as employer policies and case management standards of practice. At the beginning of the case manager/client relationship, case managers are to inform their clients that although their conversations are confidential, certain information obtained through the relationship may be disclosed to third parties including payers, service providers, and government authorities. The information shared is limited to what is necessary and relevant.

HIPAA, the Health Insurance Portability and Accountability Act, covers protected health information that is released, transferred, or divulged outside the agency. HIPAA was never intended to prevent the transfer of information. Instead, it's intent is to create national standards to protect individuals' medical records and other personal health information.

The HIPAA Privacy Rule requires healthcare providers to establish and use appropriate safeguards to protect clients' health information. This includes the transfer, storage, and destruction of records kept in any form, including records written, recorded, computerized, or stored on any other medium (U.S. Department of Health & Human Services, 2002).

Confidentially

Case managers have an obligation to maintain the confidentiality of information obtained in the course of the client-case manager relationship with few exceptions. These exceptions can vary from state to state, and by healthcare discipline (nurse, physician, social worker, psychotherapist) therefore, it is important for the case manager to be familiar with the requirements in her state.

Examples of when confidentiality can be broken:

- After receiving a written authorization from the patient
- To comply with a court order
- To report births
- To report deaths
- To report specific diseases as required by public health laws
- To report treatment of patients with a physical injury that was inflicted by non-accidental means, such as a stabbing or gunshot wound
- To report suspected neglect or exploitation of a child, elder, or resident of a long-term care facility
- When there is a duty to warn, such as to protect the patient or another party from harm

In states with Duty to Warn laws enacted, there are still differences from state to state. Some duty to warn laws are mandatory; such as reporting suspected abuse, neglect, or exploitation of children or the elderly, and some are permissive, meaning you can report without penalty but are not required to do so.

Most duty to warn laws are in place to protect the public and/or client and stem from the California courts 1976 Tarasoff v. The Regents of the University of California. The court ruled that a mental health professional, in addition to his duty to the patient, has a duty to individuals who are specifically being threatened by a patient (National Conference of State Legislatures, 2018).

***For more information, search "duty to warn" on the National Conference of State Legislatures website, www.ncsl.org

Risk Management

The goal of risk management is to reduce adverse events, decrease malpractice claims, and minimize financial loss. It can be proactive (to prevent adverse occurrences) or reactive (damage control). In both cases, the risk management process includes:

- Identifying risk or potential risk
- Calculating the probability of an adverse effect from the risk
- Estimating the impact of the adverse effect
- Control of the risk

One of the most widely used retrospective methods for improving safety is the Root Cause Analysis (RCA). RCA is a tool designed to identify what, how, and why an adverse event occurred by identifying the factors that contributed to the undesired outcome. An RCA avoids focusing on mistakes by individuals and instead focuses on errors in the system. Human error is considered inevitable, but management systems can decrease or prevent the likelihood of the adverse event occurring.

There are four steps to the RCA:

1. Data collection and reconstruction of the event in question through review of records and participant interview.

2. Causal factor charting, where information gathered is organized and analyzed by a multidisciplinary team to identify how and why the event occurred. There is rarely one causal factor, so the team should continue analyzing the information until all factors leading to the adverse outcome are identified.

3. Root cause identification, wherein the underlying reason or reasons for the causal factors in Step 2 are identified, so the problems surrounding the occurrence can be addressed.

4. Recommendation and implementation for preventing recurrence.

Legal and Regulatory Requirements Applicable to Case Management Practice

Case managers are at risk for malpractice lawsuits, even though many of them do not provide direct patient care. Patients most frequently file malpractice claims when they feel the provider was discourteous and did not take time to listen or explain the care to them. Thus, it often comes down to the basics of communication. When a patient feels the provider has listened to him, understands his situation, and has been respectful of his needs, he is very unlikely to seek legal action.

A malpractice lawsuit can arise from an act of omission (that is, failure to do something that should be done) or an act of commission (doing something that should not be done). Either of these is a breach of obligation. The plaintiff, the person bringing forth the malpractice claim, has the burden of proving two points: that the case manager was negligent and that injury resulted from the negligence.

A case manager can take several steps to reduce the risk of a malpractice lawsuit:

- Use only credentialed healthcare providers
- Offer the patient several choices for providers
- Communicate with the patient and address concerns
- Document all communications with the patient and others involved in care and decision-making
- Do not alter records
- Use written guidelines when available; if deviating from them, document justification
- Document compliance or lack of compliance with treatment plan
- Be aware of and comply with professional standards and regulations

Informed Consent

Unlike malpractice law, under tort law, a medical professional can be liable if she does not obtain informed consent before treating the patient, even if there is no injury or the patient is benefited. For example, if consent is obtained for surgery on the right eye and the surgeon performs surgery on the left eye while the patient is under anesthesia, medical battery has occurred. The surgeon can be held liable even if the patient benefited from the surgery. Other torts include negligence, false imprisonment, and assault.

The following criteria must be met for consent to be informed:

- It must include a discussion of possible side effects, risks, consequences, and benefits of treatment, medication, or procedures, including consequences or risks of stoppage of the service
- Information must be clear and easy to understand
- Information must be given verbally and in writing
- The patient must have an opportunity for questions and answers
- Consent must be self-determined; that is, it cannot be coerced or pressured by the agency or provider of services
- The client must have the capacity to make clear, competent decisions

Capacity and competence are often confused or used interchangeably. To clarify, competence follows capacity. Capacity involves a person's ability to make informed decisions and provide informed consent. Competence is a legal term and process that determines if a person has the capacity to make decisions (usually business, financial, and medical) for themself. A physician can determine capacity, but a judge will determine competence (Fink-Samnick, 2019, pp. 68-70).

Interstate Compact for Nursing

Nurse case managers must be licensed in the state where case management is being provided. Telephonic case managers who manage cases across state lines must be licensed in the state where the client is located.

The Nurse Licensure Compact gives nurses the ability to practice nursing across state lines. The nurse must be licensed in her state of residency. If the state of residency participates in the compact, she can practice in any other compact state.

Negligent Referral

Referral of a patient to a healthcare provider who is known to be unqualified is called a negligent referral. The case manager can be held liable for a negligent referral even if she is unaware that the provider is unqualified. A reasonably prudent case manager is expected to make sure the referred provider is professionally qualified and without physical or mental impairment that could result in harm to the patient.

Principal/Agent Relationship

A Principal/Agent Relationship is a relationship between a person (aka agent) and another person or entity (aka principal). The agent is authorized to act for the principal. In a healthcare setting, a doctor is an agent employed by the hospital (the principal). The doctor is authorized to act and make decisions on behalf of the hospital for patients, but the principal is responsible for the acts of the agent.

Conditions of Participation

The Centers for Medicare and Medicaid Services (CMS) has developed a set of health and safety standards that healthcare organizations must meet in order to begin and continue participation in the Medicare and Medicaid programs. These are outlined in their Conditions of Participation (CoP).

***More information can be found on the CMS website at https://www.cms.gov/Regulations-and-Guidance/Legislation/CFCsAndCoPs

The Physician Payments Sunshine Act (PPSA)

The PPSA was created to provide transparency in the relationship between physicians and manufacturers of drugs, devices, biological, and medical supplies in relation to payments and other transfers of value as well as physician ownership or investment interests in manufacturers. The act requires manufacturers to report to CMS payments or other transfers of value as well as ownership or investment interest (other than publicly traded security and mutual funds) held by a physician or immediate family member annually.

Healthcare and Disability-Related Legislation

The Americans with Disabilities Act

The Americans with Disabilities Act, or ADA, defines an individual with a disability as a person who:

- has a physical or mental impairment that substantially limits a major life activity,
- has a record or history of a substantially limiting impairment, or
- is regarded or perceived by an employer as having a substantially limiting impairment.

The ADA also protects qualified individuals with a prior drug addiction if they have been rehabilitated. However, the ADA provides that the term "individual with a disability" does not include an individual who is currently engaging in the illegal use of drugs.

Assessments are done case by case to determine if the impairment is protected under ADA. An individual, not his disability, is protected under ADA.

The ADA prohibits discrimination against people with disabilities in employment, transportation, public accommodation, communications, and governmental activities.

Employers with 15 or more employees are prohibited from discriminating against people with disabilities by Title I of the ADA. In general, the employment provisions of the ADA require:

- Equal opportunity in selecting, testing, and hiring qualified applicants with disabilities
- Job accommodation for applicants and workers with disabilities when such accommodations would not impose "undue hardship" on the employer
- Equal opportunity in promotion and benefits

An applicant with a disability, like all other applicants, must be able to meet the employer's requirements for the job, such as education, training, employment experience, skills, or licenses. In addition, an applicant with a disability must be able to perform the "essential functions" of the job either on his own or with the help of reasonable accommodation.

A job accommodation is a reasonable adjustment to a job or work environment that makes it possible for an individual with a disability to perform job duties. Determining whether to provide accommodations involves considering the required job tasks and the functional limitations of the person doing the job. An employer does not have to provide an accommodation that will cause undue hardship, defined as being significantly difficult or expensive for the employer. Accommodations may include specialized equipment (such as Dragon dictation or an elevated desk to fit a wheelchair), facility modifications (wheelchair ramps), and adjustments to work schedules or job duties, as well as a range of other creative solutions. The Job Accommodation Network (JAN) provides free consulting on workplace accommodations.

During the application/interview process, the ADA prohibits asking questions such as:

- Do you have a heart condition?
- Do you have asthma or any other difficulties breathing?

- Do you have a disability that would interfere with your ability to perform the job?
- How many days were you sick last year?
- Have you ever filed for workers' compensation? Have you ever been injured on the job?
- Have you ever been treated for mental health problems?
- What prescription drugs are you currently taking?

After a job offer is extended, an employer can ask all of the questions listed above and others that are likely to reveal the existence of a disability, as long as the same questions are asked of other applicants offered the same type of job. In other words, an employer cannot ask such questions only of those who have obvious disabilities. Similarly, an employer may require a medical examination and/or drug screen after making a job offer as long as it requires the same medical examination and/or drug screen of all applicants offered the same type of job. The employer can withdraw the job offer only if it can show that the potential employee is unable to perform the essential functions of the job (with or without reasonable accommodation), or that he poses a significant risk of causing substantial harm to himself or others.

The terms impairment, disability, and handicap are often used interchangeably, but they have very different meanings. Knowing the difference is important. Impairment refers to a problem with a structure or organ of the body. Disability is a functional limitation with regard to a particular activity. Handicap refers to a disadvantage in filling a role in life relative to peers.

Take, for example, a patient who is unable to walk after a spinal cord injury. The impairment is the inability to move his legs. The disability is the inability to walk, and the handicap is that it keeps him from fulfilling his normal role at home, work, and in the community.

Health Insurance Portability and Accountability Act (HIPAA)

HIPAA is the Health Insurance Portability and Accountability Act of 1996. Title I of the Act guarantees health insurance access, portability, and renewal; eliminates some preexisting conditions clauses; and prohibits discrimination based on health status.

Title II of HIPAA creates fraud and abuse controls, the rules for protecting the confidentiality and integrity of a client's health information, and administrative simplification. Most familiar to case managers is the safeguarding of protected health information (PHI). HIPAA covers PHI released, transferred, or divulged outside the agency. According to HIPAA, an authorization for release of PHI must be in plain, understandable language and contain a detailed description of the information to be released, the purpose of the disclosure, the individual's right to revoke the authorization, and the expiration date of the authorization. HIPAA compliance is required when using fax, phone, and Internet communications. The Act covers not only formal records, but also personal notes and billing information.

Information released under HIPAA becomes protected under the confidentiality guidelines of the organization receiving the information. The agency must have a privacy officer and safeguards to protect client records. The safeguards include electronic security of files (such as passwords) and security of work areas and destruction of files/information.

It is important to note that HIPAA does not apply to disability, auto, liability, or workers' compensation insurance and that state laws take precedence over HIPAA if they are stricter in protecting the privacy of medical records.

Occupational Safety and Health Administration (OSHA) Regulations

OSHA's mission is to assure safe and healthful workplaces by setting and enforcing standards and by providing training, outreach, education, and assistance. Employers are also required to keep their workplaces free of serious recognized hazards.

OSHA standards describe the method that employers must use to protect their employees from hazards. OSHA standards cover construction work, agriculture, maritime operations, and general industry. These standards limit the amount of hazardous chemicals workers can be exposed to, require the use of certain safe practices and equipment, and require employers to monitor hazards and keep records of workplace injuries and illnesses. Examples of OSHA standards include: to provide fall protection, prevent some infectious diseases, prevent exposure to harmful substances like asbestos, and provide training for certain dangerous jobs. A General Duty Clause also requires employers to keep the workplace free of serious recognized hazards.

OSHA covers private sector workers, not government employees. State and local government workers may be covered by an OSHA-approved state program, and federal agencies must have a safety and health program that meets the same standards as private employers. OSHA does not penalize federal agencies, but it does monitor them and respond to workers' complaints.

Family Medical Leave Act (FMLA)

The Family and Medical Leave Act (FMLA) provides eligible employees up to 12 workweeks of unpaid leave a year for specified family and medical reasons. It requires group health benefits be maintained during the leave, as if the employee continued to work. Employees are also entitled to return to their same or an equivalent job at the end of their FMLA leave.

Eligible employees are those who:

- Work for a covered employer (public agencies, including government and local schools, as well as private sector employees working for companies with 50 or more employees within a 75-mile radius of the worksite)
- Have worked 1,250 hours during the 12 months prior to the start of the leave
- Have worked for the employer for 12 months

FMLA may be taken for:

- Birth, adoption, or foster care of a child
- Care of spouse, child, or parent who has a serious health condition
- A serious health condition that makes the employee unable to perform the essential functions of his job

FMLA does not have to be taken all at once; it can be taken intermittently— taking leave in blocks of time for a single qualifying reason—or to reduce the employee's daily or weekly work schedule. The employer chooses how to count the year; calendar year, any fixed 12 months, the 12-month period measured forward, or a rolling 12 month period measured backward. This must be uniform for all employees.

The FMLA only requires that employers provide unpaid leave. However, the law permits an employee to elect or the employer to require that the employee use accrued paid vacation, sick, or family leave for some or all of the FMLA leave period. An employee must follow the employer's normal leave rules in order to substitute paid leave. When paid leave is used for an FMLA-covered reason, the leave is FMLA-protected. If the leave is unpaid, the employee must continue to pay his portion of the medical insurance that was normally deducted from his paycheck.

Pregnancy Discrimination Act

The Pregnancy Discrimination Act:

- Forbids discrimination based on pregnancy in any aspect of employment, including hiring, firing, pay, job assignments, leave, and health insurance.
- Requires health insurance provided by the employer to cover expenses for pregnancy-related conditions on the same basis as costs for other medical conditions.
- Ensures employees on leave due to pregnancy-related conditions are treated the same as other temporarily disabled employees.

Newborns' and Mothers' Health Protection Act of 1996

The Newborns' and Mothers' Health Protection Act requires that health plans and insurance issuers not restrict a mother's or newborn's benefits for a hospital stay connected to childbirth to less than 48 hours following a vaginal delivery or 96 hours following a delivery by cesarean section. However, the attending provider (who may be a physician or nurse midwife) may decide, after consulting with the mother, to discharge the mother or newborn child earlier. Incentives (either positive or negative) that could encourage an attending provider to give less than the minimum protections under the Act as described above are prohibited.

Women's Health and Cancer Rights Act of 1998

The Act requires that group health plans providing coverage for mastectomies also cover the following:

- Reconstruction of the breast that was removed by mastectomy
- Surgery and reconstruction of the other breast to make the breasts appear symmetrical
- Breast prostheses
- Complications at all stages of mastectomy, including lymphedema

Affordable Care Act (ACA)

The Affordable Care Act (ACA) has created comprehensive health insurance reforms designed to improve access, affordability, and quality in healthcare. Since its signing on March 23, 2010, the law was gradually phased in over five years and is now in full effect. The following is an overview of the key aspects of the law.

It is important to note that grandfathered individual health insurance policies bought on or before March 23, 2010, are excluded from many of the below rules.

End to pre-existing condition discrimination

Insurance companies can no longer deny coverage or charge more because of a preexisting condition. They also cannot charge more based on gender. Once insured, the insurance company cannot refuse to cover treatment for preexisting conditions.

End to arbitrary withdrawals of insurance coverage

Insurance companies can no longer drop coverage due to an honest mistake made on the application. The insurance company can rescind coverage if the application is intentionally falsified or if premium payments are not made on time, but it must give at least 30 days' notice to allow time to appeal the decision or find new coverage.

Keeps young adults covered

Adult children who cannot get coverage through their employer may remain on their parents' policies until they are 26.

Free preventative care benefits

Insurers are now required to cover a number of recommended preventive services without additional cost-sharing such as copays or deductibles. Depending on age, these preventive services include:

- Blood pressure, diabetes, and cholesterol testing
- Some cancer screenings, including mammograms and colonoscopies
- Counseling on topics such as smoking cessation, weight loss, healthy eating, treating depression, and reducing alcohol use
- Well-baby and well-child visits from birth to age 21
- Routine vaccinations
- Counseling, screening, and vaccines to ensure healthy pregnancies
- Flu and pneumonia shots

It is important to note that the health plan can require the use of network providers to receive these benefits without cost-sharing. Additionally, there may still be a fee for the office visit related to these services.

Coverage of essential health benefits

All plans offered in the individual and small group markets must cover a comprehensive package of items and services known as essential health benefits. In addition, states expanding their Medicaid programs must provide these benefits to people newly eligible for Medicaid.

Essential health benefits must include items and services within at least the following 10 categories:

- Ambulatory patient services
- Emergency services
- Hospitalization
- Maternity and newborn care
- Mental health and substance use disorder services, including behavioral health treatment (this includes counseling and psychotherapy)
- Prescription drugs
- Rehabilitative and habilitative services and devices
- Laboratory services
- Preventive and wellness services and chronic disease management
- Pediatric services, including oral and vision care (but adult dental and vision coverage are not essential health benefits)

These essential health benefits are subject to deductibles and copays. In addition, self-funded employer plans and grandfathered plans are not required to cover these benefits.

End to dollar limits on care

The ACA bans annual and lifetime dollar limits on most covered health benefits. In the past, people with cancer or other illnesses could lose their insurance coverage when their healthcare expenses reached the dollar limit on their policy. It is important to note that there are some exceptions to this ban on limits—for example, grandfathered individual plans are not required to follow the rules on annual limits—and plans can put an annual dollar limit and a lifetime dollar limit on spending for healthcare services that are not essential health benefits.

Requires Mental Health Coverage

The Affordable Care Act requires that most individual and small employer health insurance plans, including all plans offered through the Health Insurance Marketplace, cover mental health and substance use disorder services. Also required are rehabilitative and habilitative services that can help support people with behavioral health challenges.

Paying physicians based on value not volume

A provision that took effect in 2015 ties physician Medicare payments to the quality of care they provide. Medicare payments will be modified so that physicians who provide higher value care will receive higher payments than those who provide lower quality care (U.S. Department of Health & Human Services, 2019).

Linking payment to quality outcomes

The ACA established a hospital Value-Based Purchasing program (VBP) in traditional Medicare. This program offers financial incentives to hospitals to improve the quality of care. It is based on either: 1) how well they perform on each measure compared to other hospitals, or 2) how much they improved their own performance on each measure compared to their performance during a prior baseline period. Hospital performance is required to be publicly reported, beginning with measures relating to heart attacks, heart failure, pneumonia, surgical care, healthcare-associated infections, and patients' perception of care.

Hospital Readmission Reduction Program

The ACA authorizes Medicare to reduce payments to acute care hospitals with excess readmissions that are paid under CMS's Inpatient Prospective Payment System (IPPS). Excess readmissions are measured by a ratio, by dividing a hospital's number of "predicted" 30-day readmissions for heart attack, heart failure, pneumonia, hip/knee replacement, and COPD, by the number that would be "expected," based on an average hospital with similar patients. A ratio greater than one indicates excess readmissions.

The ACA also identifies ways to improve the often-fragmented healthcare system, such as the patient-centered medical home and the accountable care organization. Both of these rely on care coordination as a central pillar of their success.

**More information on these models of care can be found in the chapter Delivery and Reimbursement Methods under Models of Care.

Impact for Case Management

The ACA provides many incentives to improve quality, coordinate care, and decrease costs—all areas where case managers are well-positioned to take the lead. The impact case managers can have in this new value-driven care world are tremendous. Case management functions, such as assessing, planning, educating, discharge planning, care transitioning, care coordination, and monitoring, are key to meeting the savings benchmarks and quality performance standards outlined in the ACA.

HITECH Act

The American Reinvestment & Recovery Act (ARRA) was enacted on February 17, 2009. ARRA includes many measures aimed at modernizing our nation's infrastructure, one of which is the "Health Information Technology for Economic and Clinical Health (HITECH) Act." The HITECH Act included the concept of electronic health records–meaningful use [EHR-MU], an effort led by CMS and the Office of the National Coordinator for Health IT (ONC). In April of 2018, CMS renamed EHR-MU (aka Meaningful Use) to Public Health and Promoting Interoperability Programs (Centers for Disease Control and Prevention, 2019).

HITECH made the meaningful use of interoperable electronic health records throughout the United States healthcare delivery system a critical national goal.

Meaningful Use required the use of certified EHR technology in a meaningful manner (for example electronic prescribing). Additional accomplishments of Meaningful Use were the use of certified EHR technology for the electronic exchange of health information to improve the quality of healthcare and the use of certified EHR technology to submit clinical quality measures.

In changing the name to Public Health and Promoting Interoperability Programs, CMS has moved the programs beyond the existing requirement of meaningful use to a new phase of EHR measurement with an increased focus on interoperability and improving patient access to health information.

There are specific objectives that eligible professionals (EPs) and hospitals must achieve to qualify for Medicare and Medicaid Promoting Interoperability Programs incentives (known as the EHR Incentive Programs prior to April 2018). The following is a closer look at two of the objectives and their clinical importance (Centers for Disease Control and Prevention, 2019).

Electronic Exchanges of Summary of Care

Objective

EPs who transition their patients to another setting of care or provider of care, or refer their patients to another provider of care, should provide a summary care record for each transition of care or referral. For this objective, the term "transition of care" is defined as the movement of a patient from one setting of care (e.g., hospital, ambulatory primary care practice, specialty care practice, long-term care, home health care, or rehabilitation facility) to another. A summary of care record must include the following elements:

- Patient name
- Referring or transitioning provider's name and office contact information
- Procedures
- Encounter diagnosis
- Immunizations
- Laboratory test results
- Vital signs (height, weight, blood pressure, BMI)
- Smoking status
- Functional status, including activities of daily living, cognitive and disability status
- Demographic information (preferred language, sex, race, ethnicity, date of birth)
- Care plan field (at a minimum, the following components must be included: problem-focus of the care plan, goal-target outcome, and any instructions that the provider has given to the patient)
- Care team, including the primary care provider of record and any additional known care team members beyond the referring or transitioning provider and the receiving provider
- Reason for the referral
- Current problem list (at minimum, a list of current, active, and historical diagnoses, but the problem list is not limited to diagnoses)
- Current medication list
- Current medication allergy list

Clinical importance

A transition of care summary, also known as a discharge summary in some circumstances, provides essential clinical information for the receiving care team and helps organize final clinical and administrative activities for the transferring care team. This summary helps ensure the coordination and continuity of healthcare as patients transfer between different locations or different levels of care within the same location. This document improves transitions and discharges, communication among providers, and cross-setting relationships, which can improve care quality and safety.

E-Prescribing (eRx)

Objective

To generate and transmit permissible prescriptions electronically.

Definitions of terms:

> Permissible Prescriptions – This refers to the current restrictions established by the Department of Justice on electronic prescribing for controlled substances in Schedule II-V. Any prescription not subject to these restrictions would be permissible.

> Prescription – The authorization by an EP to a pharmacist to dispense a drug that the pharmacist would not dispense to the patient without such authorization.

Clinical importance

Electronic prescribing is a fast, efficient way to write/reorder and transmit prescriptions. ERx has pre-set fields, so all required information is entered and automatically stored in the patient's record for easy review during follow-up visits or for transitions to other providers. E-Prescribing increases overall patient satisfaction because the prescriptions can be automatically transmitted to a pharmacy of preference. Electronic systems also provide guided dose algorithms to assist providers. Providers may also query the patient's health plan formulary to ensure the drug selected is covered, which may reduce costs to the patient.

Self-care, Safety, and Well-being as a Professional

In the course of their work, case managers are routinely in contact with multiple stakeholders including patients, their families, physicians, employers, insurance companies, and vendors, all of whom may have their own agendas and potentially competing priorities. Often case managers are asked to do more with less, which can add to the stress and overwhelm of their job.

Add to this the feeling of powerlessness related to hierarchical power structures, ineffective or obstructive policies, dysfunctional communication, lack of resources, and other issues beyond their control, and you have moral distress (Epstein, 2009, pp. 330-342). Moral distress is defined as knowing the right thing to do, but institutional constraints make it nearly impossible to pursue the right course of action (Jameton, 1984).

The ability to take charge of moral distress is critical to a case manager's wellness and long-term sustainability in the workforce. Obtaining support and validation from colleagues and mentors will empower your efforts (Fink-Samnick, 2019, pp. 68–70). This is one of the many reasons why professional organizations play an important role in professional case management. They offer a network of colleagues and mentors to consult and collaborate with outside of the organization the case manager is employed by, who can bring a fresh perspective and sense of camaraderie.

Burnout, closely related to moral distress, is a prolonged response to chronic emotional and interpersonal stressors on the job evidenced by exhaustion, cynicism, and inefficacy (Maslach et al., 2001). One step case managers can take to avoid burnout is to set boundaries with clients and stakeholders. This involves defining clear expectations of the case manager's roles and responsibilities along with that of each stakeholder. It can also include methods and times of communication, appropriate response times, and other boundaries that help the case manager to avoid burnout.

It is common that, in the course of caring for everyone else, a case manager will neglect to care for themself. Case managers should actively look after their own well-being so they can effectively support their clients. Although self-care is a personal matter that everyone approaches differently, there are some fundamental components, such as lowering stress, engaging in healthy practices, and participating in activities that give energy. Ways to engage in self-care include:

- Exercising regularly
- Eating a well-balanced diet
- Developing a regular sleep routine and getting adequate sleep
- Engaging in hobbies or interests
- Fostering positive relationships
- Taking breaks throughout the day, including a lunch break
- Learning to say no
- Taking time to relax

Self-care is a daily, long-term activity that takes practice. When case management work gets overwhelming, it's important to keep things in perspective, ask for help, and embrace change.

BONUS

The CCM exam can be intimidating to many case managers, but there are a few simple test taking strategies I can teach you that will significantly increase your chances of passing the first time. I recorded a video to review these with you. You can access it at CCMcertificationMadeEasy.com

References

Centers for Disease Control and Prevention. (n.d.). *Public Health and Promoting Interoperability Programs (formerly, known as Electronic Health Records Meaningful Use).* https://www.cdc.gov/ehrmeaningfuluse/introduction.html

Commission for Case Management Certification. (2017). *Glossary of terms.* https://ccmcertification.org/get-certified/exam-study-materials/ccmc-glossary

Epstein, E.G., & Hamric, A.B. (2009, Winter). Moral distress, moral residue, and the crescendo effect. J Clin Ethics. 2009;20:330–342.

Fink-Samnick, E. (2019). The essential guide to interprofessional ethics in healthcare case management. Hcpro.

Jameton, A. (1984). Nursing practice: The ethical issues. Prentice-Hall.

Maslach, C., Schaufeli, W. B., & Leiter, M. P. (2001). Job burnout. Annual Review of Psychology, 52(1), 397–422. https://doi.org/10.1146/annurev.psych.52.1.397

National Conference of State Legislatures. (2018, October 12). *Mental health professionals' duty to warn.* https://www.ncsl.org/research/health/mental-health-professionals-duty-to-warn.aspx

U.S. Department of Health & Human Services. (2019, February 25). *Does the Affordable Care Act cover individuals with mental health problems?* https://www.hhs.gov/answers/affordable-care-act/does-the-aca-cover-individuals-with-mental-health-problems/index.html

U.S. Department of Health & Human Services. (2013, July 26). *What does HIPAA privacy rule do?* https://www.hhs.gov/hipaa/for-individuals/faq/187/what-does-the-hipaa-privacy-rule-do/index.html

<<<< >>>>

Test Your Knowledge On Ethical, Legal, and Practice Standards

1. Case Management's ethical principles are:

    A. Autonomy, beneficence, fidelity, justice, malfeasance

    B. Advocacy, fidelity, justice, non-malfeasance, veracity

    C. Autonomy, beneficence, fidelity, justice, non-malfeasance

    D. Advocacy, beneficence, fidelity, justice, non-malfeasance

2. Board-certified case managers must honor all of the following except:

    A. Federal, state, and local laws regarding client privacy and confidentiality

    B. Employer policies and procedures

    C. Case Management Standards of Practice

    D. Their client's goals

3. Documentation is important for all of the following except:

    A. Assist in clinical management

    B. Justifies interventions and expenses

    C. Defense in claims of negligence

    D. Direct care for clients

4. Fidelity refers to the ethical principle that directs case managers to:

    A. Assure equity across treatment

    B. Keep commitments or promises

    C. Promote privacy and confidentiality

    D. Maintain honesty in interactions

5. Juggling competing professional values where there is no right answer refers to:

A. Professional Bias

B. Moral Distress

C. Ethical dilemmas

D. Professional Resilience

6. To be an ethical dilemma, all of the following conditions must be present, except:

A. A decision for the case manager to make on the job

B. Different correct courses of action to choose from

C. Compromising of an ethical principle through any presenting action

D. Conflict with a personal value

7. Which of the following elements is not true of the Americans with Disabilities Act (ADA)?

A. Protects qualified individuals with a prior drug addiction if they have been rehabilitated

B. Prohibits discrimination against people with disabilities in employment

C. Applies to employers with 10 or more employees.

D. Allows for reasonable job accommodations to be provided

8. The Agency responsible for assuring safe and healthful workplaces is:

A. The Joint Commission

B. The Occupational Safety and Health Administration

C. The Commission for Case Manager Certification

D. The National Commission for Quality Assurance

9. Which Act may the case manager reference when working with a client with breast cancer who is being denied reconstructive surgery?

    A. The Americans With Disabilities Act

    B. The Women's Health and Cancer Rights Act

    C. The Affordable Care Act

    D. Mental Health Parity Act

10. Client confidentiality can be broken:

    A. When there is a duty to warn in order to protect a patient or another person

    B. When the case manager needs information

    C. Where there is a dispute with the insurance company

    D. When a client wants to start an experimental protocol

11. Which document appoints someone to make healthcare decisions on behalf of the client if the client is not able to make their own decisions?

    A. Living Will

    B. Viatical Settlement

    C. Healthcare Durable Power of Attorney

    D. The American with Disabilities Act

12. Meaningful Use refers to:

    A. A requirement for patient care planning under URAC

    B. A requirement for case management accreditation under the National Committee for Quality Assurance

    C. A CMS program that awards incentives for using certified Electronic Health Records

D. A requirement for healthcare organizations under HIPAA

13. What is the term when the case manager has a responsibility toward a third party other than the client (e.g., case manager/payer/client or case manager/ employer/client)?

A. Use of Professional Self

B. Dual relationship

C. Moral imperative

D. Clinical Necessity

14. Which of the following is not true regarding Risk Management?

A. Identifies risk or potential risk

B. Can use Root Cause Analysis

C. Defines the clear cause of adverse effects

D. Is directly addressed in the professional case management standards

15. Case managers advocate for the patient and payer, but if a conflict arises the priority is:

A. The payer

B. The decision is deferred to the PCP

C. Neither, this is an ethical dilemma

D. The patient

Answer Key

1. Answer: C

   Rationale: Autonomy, beneficence, fidelity, justice, non-malfeasance are the seminal ethical principles for case managers to guide the practice of case management.

   Refer to: Subdomain–Ethics Related to Care Delivery.

2. Answer: D

   Rationale: Client's goals should be honored but if not safe, case managers need to redirect those goals or inform clients of risk.

   Refer to: Subdomain–Standards of Practice.

3. Answer: D

   Rationale: Case Managers do not direct care for their clients.

   Refer to: Subdomain–Case Recording and Documentation.

4. Answer: B

   Rationale: Fidelity refers to follow-through, keeping commitments, and promises A, C or D do not apply to the ethical term of Fidelity.

   Refer to: CCMC Glossary of Terms.

5. Answer: C

   Rationale: Ethical dilemmas arise when there is no right answer to a situation. The case manager must always err on the side of the patient when an ethical dilemma arises.

   Refer to: Subdomain–Ethics Related to Care Delivery.

6. Answer: D

   Rationale: Ethical dilemmas occur when there is no "right" answer or decision. A, B, and C reflect the three conditions that must be present for an ethical dilemma to be identified. D may create a personal dilemma but does not meet the criteria for an ethical dilemma.

Refer to: Subdomain–Ethics Related to Professional Practice.

7. Answer: C

Rationale: Employers with 15 or more employees must comply with the Americans with Disability Act, ADA

Refer to: Subdomain–Healthcare and Disability Related Legislation.

8. Answer: B

Rationale: Safe workplaces are important for employers and employees. OSHA is the organization that is set up to set safety policies to help keep workplaces safe.

Refer to: Subdomain–Healthcare and Disability Related Legislation.

9. Answer: B

Rationale: The Women's Health and Cancer Rights Act of 1998 requires that group health plans providing coverage for mastectomies also provide coverage for reconstruction, surgery, prosthesis, and complications related to the mastectomy.

Refer to: Subdomain–Healthcare and Disability Related Legislation.

10. Answer: A

Rationale: Confidentiality can be broken in a few situations. When there is a duty to warn is one of the situations which allows for confidentiality to be broken.

Refer to: Subdomain–Privacy and Confidentiality.

11. Answer: C

Rationale: The healthcare power of attorney is the document that will appoint someone to make healthcare decisions in case a person is unable to do so themself.

Refer to: Subdomain–Ethics Related to Care Delivery.

12. Answer: C

Rationale: Meaningful use was part of the HITECH Act concept of electronic health records. HITECH proposed the meaningful use of interoperable electronic health records throughout the United States healthcare delivery system as a critical national goal.

Refer to: Subdomain–Healthcare and Disability Related Legislation.

13. Answer: B

Rationale: A dual relationship exists when the case manager has responsibilities toward a third party other than the client. (e.g., client/employer, client/provider, client/payer)

Refer to: CCMC Glossary of Terms.

14. Answer: D

Rationale: Professional case management standards do not directly address Risk Management.

Refer to: CMSA Standards of Practice.

15. Answer: D

Rationale: Case managers advocate for both the client and the payer to facilitate positive outcomes for the client, the interprofessional healthcare team, and the payer. However, if a conflict arises, the needs of the client must be the number one priority.

Refer to: CMSA Standards of Practice.

Appendix

Practice Test

1. Which of the following statements is true regarding the Social Determinants of Health?

    A. Case managers are not concerned with the Social Determinants of Health as they are not medical issues.

    B. They include age, race, and gender.

    C. The social determinants of health are the factors that affect health outside of the hospital and doctor's office and include but are not limited to housing, social services, geographical location, and education.

    D. They only affect individuals below the poverty level.

2. Which case management step classifies patients into a low, moderate, or high category?

    A. Assessing

    B. Case planning

    C. Evaluation

    D. Stratifying risk

3. Appropriate steps the case manager can take to help prevent burnout and moral distress include all of the following except:

    A. Joining a professional organization for peer support

    B. Setting appropriate boundaries with clients and employer

    C. Venting about problem clients on social media

    D. Engage in self-care activities

4. The purpose of the Cost-Benefit Report can include all of the following except:

    A. To formally document monetary savings related to case management involvement

    B. To justify more costly intervention

    C. Document improvement in quality directly related to case management intervention

    D. To demonstrate hard cost savings

5. Which example below suggests an adaptive family?

    A. Giving the patient any kind of food he/she wants to cheer them up

B. Rotating commitments of assistance among local family members

C. One family member responsible for all aspects of assistance

D. Communication is limited to certain family members

6. An example of hard cost savings is:

A. Decrease in length of stay because the case manager alerted the doctor the patient was stable and a bed was ready in the step-down unit.

B. Avoidance of re-admission

C. Prevention of complication following surgery

D. Avoidance of Emergency Department Visits

7. A disability that is caused by either a work-related injury or occupational illness resulting in some form of permanent impairment that makes a worker unable to perform at their full capacity is:

A. Permanent Partial Disability Benefit

B. Permanent Partial Disability (PPD)

C. Permanent Total Disability

D. Physical Disability

8. The Functional Capacity Evaluation (FCE) is used to do all of the following except:

A. Assess an individual's physical capacities.

B. Assess an individual's functional abilities.

C. Establish the physical level of work an individual can perform.

D. Assess the individual's mental capacities.

9. Clients receiving any treatment, especially those experimental must:

A. Allow family input toward decision-making

B. Give informed consent

C. Discuss with all members of the treatment team

D. Try other treatment options first

10. A patient has an insurance plan with a $250 deductible for in-network care. They also have a copay of $25 per visit. The charge for services with an in-network provider is $400. The patient has satisfied $200 of this year's deductible. What is the patient's financial responsibility for this visit?

    A. $300
    B. $75
    C. $50
    D. $100

11. Dual diagnosis refers to:

    A. Clients with coexisting substance use and mental illness meeting the criteria for diagnosis by the Diagnostic and Statistical Manual of Mental Disorders (DSM-5)
    B. Clients with coexisting substance abuse disorders and mental illness meeting the criteria for diagnosis by the Diagnostic and Statistical Manual of Mental Disorders (DSM-5)
    C. Clients with coexisting heart disease and diabetes
    D. Clients with Post Traumatic Stress Disorder (PTSD) and substance abuse disorder

12. A program for injured workers that focuses on work endurance and uses real or simulated job tasks and duties with the ultimate goal of returning the worker to gainful employment is:

    A. Work conditioning
    B. Work hardening
    C. Supported employment
    D. Workers' Compensation

13. Individuals who do not identify with the gender assigned at birth often have barriers to healthcare that can include all of the following except:

    A. Name on the insurance card and medical records do not match the identified name
    B. Denial of medically necessary treatment and preventive care if the sex on file with insurance does not match the anatomy
    C. Lack of healthcare providers trained in transgender medical and behavioral healthcare
    D. Job discrimination

14. Which of the following about accreditation is incorrect?

    A. Accreditation is a standardized program for evaluating healthcare organizations to ensure a specified level of quality.

    B. Accreditation is a mandatory process for evaluating healthcare organizations to ensure a minimum standard of quality is met.

    C. Accreditation involves a voluntary survey process that assesses the healthcare organization's compliance with standards.

    D. Accreditation is regarded as one of the key benchmarks for measuring the quality of an organization.

15. The legal document that directs healthcare, specifically which treatments should be withheld, or withdrawing life support measures is:

    A. Medical power of attorney

    B. Living will

    C. Advance directive

    D. Do not resuscitate order

16. Which term defines a person having the skills and training that are commonly necessary in the labor market to be gainfully employed on a reasonably continuous basis when considering the person's age, education, experience, physical, and mental capacities due to industrial injury or disease?

    A. Employability

    B. Fitness for Duty

    C. Able-Bodied

    D. Professional

17. For case managers required to complete patient care reports, the frequency of patient's reports can vary but should always be done:

    A. Then changes occur with the patient

    B. At case closure

    C. When cost savings are realized

    D. When the insurance company requests an update

18. Case Management's ethical principles are:

    A. Autonomy, beneficence, fidelity, justice, malfeasance

    B. Advocacy, fidelity, justice, non-malfeasance, veracity

    C. Autonomy, beneficence, fidelity, justice, non-malfeasance

    D. Advocacy, beneficence, fidelity, justice, non-malfeasance

19. The client statement of "I'm not ready to give up beer yet but I am thinking I need to do this soon." is an example of which stage of Behavioral Change?

    A. Contemplative

    B. Preparation

    C. Pre-Contemplative

    D. Action

20. The workers' compensation system is administered by:

    A. State statutes

    B. The federal government

    C. Place of employment

    D. Individual insurance brokers

21. All of the following are ways the case manager can foster and encourage self-efficacy in the client, except:

    A. Facilitating goal setting that will promote mastery by helping the client create small, attainable goals

    B. Assisting the client to reach optimal physical and psychological function by making referrals as needed

    C. Assessing for barriers to compliance with the care plan

    D. Providing affirmation, motivation, and encouragement

22. Raising the height of a desk to provide access for a wheelchair is an example of a:

    A. Work adjustment

    B. Job restructuring

    C. Job accommodation

    D. Building Modification

23. Reports case managers can use to demonstrate their value include all of the following except:

    A. Quality Improvement Reports

    B. Cost benefits of case management services

    C. Incident Reports

    D. Justification to continue interventions

24. The main objective of the planning step is to:

    A. Develop an individualized case management plan

    B. Gather input from the patient and caregiver

    C. Develop Short term goals

    D. Prioritize goals

25. Which of the following psychiatric disabilities is not protected by the Americans with Disabilities Act?

    A. Post-traumatic stress syndrome

    B. Kleptomania

    C. Depression

    D. Bipolar disorder

26. All of the following are health benefits of spirituality except:

    A. Spiritual practices tend to improve coping skills and provide optimism and hope

    B. Spiritual practices can positively influence immune, cardiovascular, and hormonal systems

    C. Decreased depression and anxiety

    D. Increased compliance with a treatment plan by clients who consider themselves spiritual

27. Which program exists for clients age 18-64 who want to return to work and currently receive Social Security Disability based on disability under the Social Security Disability Insurance program or under the Supplemental Security Income Program?

    A. Americans With Disability Act

B. Ticket to Work Program

C. Job Development Program

D. Self Determination Act

28. Which of the following would be most appropriate to conduct to determine the requirements and duties of a given job including the skills and competencies needed to perform the job?

A. Job analysis

B. Job adjustment

C. Vocational assessment

D. Vocational Testing

29. Which tool would not be viewed as a healthcare analytic tool to identify at-risk individuals who may benefit from case management services?

A. Health Risk Assessment

B. Predictive Modeling

C. Adjusted Clinical Groups

D. Case Management Survey

30. A patient with traditional Medicare is discharged from the hospital following a 50-day stay. The patient is readmitted one month later. The second admission is:

A. A new benefit period

B. The same benefit period

C. Immediately subject to a daily co-pay

D. A non-covered stay

31. Client Engagement is best demonstrated by the following actions:

A. Daily monitoring and recording of weight and vital signs

B. Delay in contacting the home health agency to report equipment is not working

C. Frequent calls to the cardiologist to report minor changes in weight.

D. Lack of follow-through due to cognitive deficits

32. The ADA requires employers to provide reasonable accommodations for qualified applicants or employees with disabilities unless doing so would cause undue hardship for the employer. Undue hardship can refer to all of the following except:

    A. Accommodations that cause financial difficulty

    B. Accommodations that are disruptive to the workplace

    C. Accommodations that fundamentally change the operation of the business

    D. Accommodations that cost more than 20% of the employee's annual salary

33. In the area of workers' compensation, the person who investigates claims by interviewing the claimant and other involved parties (e.g., employers and witnesses), reviews related records, and assures that medical care is available to the worker as needed based on the injury or occupational illness is known as:

    A. Claims Adjuster

    B. Claimant

    C. Vocational Counselor

    D. Attorney

34. Health Maintenance Organizations (HMOs) and Exclusive Provider Organizations (EPOs) are examples of:

    A. Managed care

    B. Workers' compensation

    C. Self-funded plans

    D. Prospective payment systems

35. The case manager changes the medical record by adding a 0 to a lab value so that the patient meets criteria for additional inpatient days and the hospital is paid. This is:

    A. Advocacy

    B. Fraud

    C. Acceptable as a zero holds no value and therefore nothing was done

    D. Financial stewardship

36. This analysis reveals whether the benefits of an action, intervention, service, or treatment outweigh the cost, and by how much, so that the involved party is able to make the appropriate decision(s):

A. Job Analysis

B. Data analysis

C. Cost-benefit analysis

D. Root cause analysis

37. Conflict Resolution strategies include all of the following except:

A. Accommodation

B. Negotiation

C. Collaboration

D. Family Coordination

38. The Instrumental Activities of Daily Living (IADL) tool includes assessment of all of the following except:

A. Shopping

B. Ability to use the telephone

C. Ability to navigate stairs

D. Ability to handle finances

39. The goal for case managers who specialize in the area of workers' compensation is to:

A. Ensure care is coordinated to avoid duplication and fragmentation of care and contain costs

B. Return the injured worker to gainful employment

C. Limit medical care to the work-related injury

D. Educate the employer on the importance of improving workplace safety

40. A quantifiable metric used to measure quality is:

A. Quality monitoring

B. A quality indicator

C. Risk management

D. A quality rating

41. According to The American Psychiatric Association's Diagnostic and Statistical Manual of Mental Disorders, 5th Edition (DSM-5), substance abuse:

A. Does not include alcohol, over the counter drugs, or prescription drugs

B. Includes anyone who uses illegal substances in any amount

C. Is a maladaptive pattern of substance use leading to clinically significant impairment or distress

D. Substance abuse is not addressed as it is not considered a mental disorder

42. Board-certified case managers are not to:

A. Make decisions for their clients based on the best evidence available.

B. Participate in ongoing professional development.

C. Perform comprehensive assessments to identify needs.

D. Be knowledgeable about and act in accordance with all laws related to their scope of practice

43. Performance improvement measures of structure include:

A. The number of qualified staff, accreditation status, and access to technologies

B. Accreditation status, outcomes, and processes

C. Access to technologies, outcomes, and processes

D. Mortality rates, percentage of clients screened for breast cancer

44. Under the Americans with Disabilities Act, which of the following questions can't be asked in an interview?

A. What was your previous pay?

B. What strengths do you bring to this position?

C. What medical issues could impact your performance?

D. Have you ever been convicted of a felony?

45. The case management assessment can be done in person or telephonically and should include information primarily from the:

A. Client

B. Pharmacist

C. Neighbors

D. Employee

46. By working with her hospital's quality assurance team toward improving quality care outcomes for their patient population, the case manager is demonstrating which ethical principle?

    A. Quality Assurance (QA)

    B. Quality Improvement (QI)

    C. Fidelity

    D. Non-Maleficence

47. Which of the following statements is true regarding spirituality?

    A. Spirituality is separate from religion and therefore spiritual beliefs can be challenged with the patient

    B. Religious beliefs and spiritual beliefs are the same

    C. The client's spiritual beliefs often impact the choices clients make regarding their healthcare

    D. The topic of spirituality should not be introduced by the case manager, but they may continue the conversation if brought up by the client.

48. A Life Care Plan would be most appropriate for which of the following?

    A. A hospice patient

    B. A patient with a new terminal diagnosis

    C. A client enrolling in case management

    D. A client with a traumatic brain injury (TBI) resulting in cognitive and physical deficits that require around the clock supervision

49. The purpose of managed care is to:

    A. Improve access to care

    B. Limit access to care

    C. Maintain quality while managing costs

    D. Provide care while limiting choice

50. Health Literacy Instruments are available to assist in the assessment of health literacy, which of the following is an established instrument?

    A. Rancho Los Amigos Scale of Cognitive Functioning

B. The Newest Vital Sign

C. Glasgow Coma Score (GCS)

D. Clinical Health Risk Assessment (HRA)

51. Which step of the case management process focuses on assessing the effectiveness of the case management plan?

A. Post transition communication

B. Transitional planning

C. Assessing

D. Evaluating outcomes

52. The health risk assessment (HRA) is a useful tool used to assess a patient's health status, risk of negative health outcomes, and readiness to change certain behaviors but it has limitations, which include all of the following except:

A. It is time-consuming as it requires significant 1:1 time to administer

B. Its reliance on the patient's recall can make it unreliable

C. Clients may be reluctant to report socially unacceptable behaviors such as smoking or alcohol use

D. Language, culture, and literacy levels can affect the results

53. Using verbal insults, intimidation, or threats to withhold food as a means of getting an elderly patient to take their medication are examples of:

A. Coercion

B. Physical abuse

C. Psychological abuse

D. Acceptable methods to persuade the patient to take their medication

54. What is the purpose of pharmacy benefit management?

A. Provide prescription medication in the most cost-effective manner

B. Provide medication reconciliation services

C. Prevent opioid abuse

D. Assure patient adherence

55. The case manager is working with a client in a smoking cessation program. The client makes the statement, "I have not had a cigarette in 4 months." The client is in which stage of change?

    A. Maintenance

    B. Action

    C. Preparation

    D. Completed

56. Which of the following statements regarding substance use rehabilitation is incorrect?

    A. Detoxification should be followed by ongoing drug addiction treatment

    B. Community-based programs such as Alcoholics Anonymous and Narcotics Anonymous have been found to be the most successful in treating substance abuse

    C. Inpatient hospitalization for substance abuse is not usually the preferred method of treatment

    D. Detoxification alone addresses the psychological, social, and behavioral problems associated with addiction and therefore if done correctly will produce the lasting behavioral change necessary for recovery

57. Which best defines the role of an advocate?

    A. Educating the client, family regarding treatment options

    B. Collaborating with patient and family

    C. Ensuring the client's needs are priority

    D. Speaking on the behalf of the client and promoting their cause when needed

58. The Medicare hospice benefit:

    A. Is provided under Part A

    B. Covers all patient prescriptions

    C. Is limited to 90 days

    D. Has a $50 deductible

59. What group provides a wide array of services available in the community for those 60 years and older?

    A. Area Agency on Aging

B. The Lions Society

C. Veterans of Foreign Wars

D. Meals on Wheels

60. A case manager who mainly focuses on vocational/return to work activities works in what area of case management?

A. University clinics

B. Healthcare centers

C. Acute rehabilitation

D. Workers' compensation

61. When researching a rehabilitation facility for a client, which accreditation would the case manager look for?

A. Utilization Review Accreditation Commission (URAC)

B. National Committee for Quality Assurance (NCQA)

C. American Association of Retired Persons (AARP)

D. Commission on Accreditation of Rehabilitation Facilities (CARF)

62. To qualify for home care under Medicare, a patient must be:

A. Homebound and require assistance with ADLs

B. Homebound and require full-time nursing

C. Homebound and require skilled services

D. Homebound and require services associated with a hospital or SNF stay

63. The Minnesota Multiphasic Personality Inventory (MMPI) is:

A. A psychological test that assesses personality traits and psychopathology

B. Used to measure the patient's level of depression

C. A brief assessment used to screen for cognitive impairment and related dementia

D. To measure the level of coma in the acute phase of an injury

64. A woman is hospitalized for a c-section. She is covered by her own employer's health plan and as a dependent on her husband's employer's health plan. According to COB, which health plan pays first?

A. Family Medical Leave Act (FMLA)

B. Her short term disability policy

C. Her employee health plan

D. Her husband's employee health plan

65. Achieving optimal outcomes, quality of care, appropriate use of services and resources, optimum health and functioning for the client and client's knowledge of disease are examples of:

A. Negotiation techniques

B. Management of chronic conditions

C. Improving patient adherence

D. Goals and objectives of case management

66. Mrs. Smith has been receiving Social Security Disability Income for 7 years. She will be turning 65 in 2 months. Once she turns 65 her SSDI will:

A. Be discontinued

B. Decrease

C. Increase

D. Convert to Social Security Income

67. Benchmarking aids a healthcare organization to assess:

A. How they perform against their peers and where improvement might be pursued

B. Their share of the marketplace in relation to their competitors'

C. If they have reached their goals

D. Their strengths for marketing purposes

68. The Americans with Disabilities Act defines a disability as all of the following except:

A. Is unable to work despite recovering from an injury/illness

B. Has a physical or mental impairment that substantially limits a major life activity

C. Has a record or history of a substantially limiting impairment

D. Is regarded or perceived by an employer as having a substantially limited activity

69. Individuals at highest risk for low health literacy which can lead to uncontrolled chronic conditions, less frequent use of preventive services, increased likelihood of using medications incorrectly, and higher rates of hospitalization and emergency department use include all of the following except:

    A. Older adults

    B. Those having less than a 4-year college education

    C. Those speaking English as their second language

    D. Those whose income is at or below the poverty level

70. Which of the following does not reflect a potential conflict of interest for case managers?

    A. A case manager is employed at a home health agency and a Long Term Acute Care facility

    B. A Director of Case Management writes industry-focused journal articles

    C. A case manager is employed at a hospital and a home health agency

    D. A case management consultant sits on the Board of Directors for a professional association to solicit business

71. The Americans with Disabilities Act protects individuals with drug addiction in which of the following employment situations?

    A. The individual is applying for employment and has active drug use

    B. The individual is employed, found positive for drug use but has agreed to start a rehabilitation program

    C. An applicant who is not qualified for the position but successfully completed a drug rehabilitation program

    D. An employee with a recently found history of drug use, who has been successfully rehabbed and is no longer using drugs

72. Case Management promotes what kind of outcomes?

    A. Those that can be obtained for the lowest cost

    B. Quality and cost-efficient outcomes

    C. Patient determined outcomes

    D. Provider recommended outcomes

73. Self-efficacy plays a major role in the client's outcome. The more self-efficacy a client possesses, the more likely he or she will persevere when obstacles arise. Self-efficacy is:

    A. One's belief in his or her own ability to succeed

    B. One's ability to advocate for himself or herself

    C. One's feeling of power or control of a situation

    D. One's ability to provide for their physical needs such as food, clothing, and shelter

74. Which of the following statements regarding performance improvement is correct?

    A. Performance improvement is always prospective

    B. Performance improvement is designed to attribute blame

    C. Performance improvement is always retrospective

    D. Performance improvement can focus on process, structure, and/or outcomes

75. Mrs. K, a 68-year-old retired lawyer, has been in treatment for cancer off and on for 5 years. During her most recent recurrence, she has gone through 3 lines of chemo with no success. Her performance scores are low and her current prognosis is 4-6 months. There is a clinical trial that she qualifies for but it is a double-blind phase I and unlikely to reverse her disease progression. Mrs. K would like to enter the clinical trial and begin hospice. Her doctor responds:

    A. You cannot choose curative treatment and hospice

    B. You can do both because a clinical trial is not a standard treatment

    C. Clinical trials are not available to Medicare patients

    D. This is a phase I trial and phase I clinical trials are not covered by Medicare

76. What are two common negotiation strategies?

    A. Collaboration and compromise

    B. Aggressive and cooperative

    C. Intimidation and discussion

    D. Acceptable and damaging

77. Quality assurance is:

    A. A predetermined measure for assessing quality

B. A government agency whose purpose is to ensure that Medicare recipients receive quality care

C. An array of techniques and methods used to collect and analyze data

D. The use of activities and programs to monitor, prevent, and correct quality deficiencies and ensure quality

78. Patient Self Determination Act (PSDA) ensures which important documents are recognized by hospitals?

A. Power of Attorney

B. Informed Consent

C. End of life documents such as a Living Will and Durable Power of Attorney for Healthcare

D. HIPAA Release Form

79. Which of the following pays for medical care for work-related injuries?

A. Short Term Disability

B. Long Term Disability

C. Workers' Compensation

D. Employee health benefit

80. Health coaching is for:

A. Clients who suffer from a chronic disease

B. Clients who want to prevent disease

C. Caregivers of patients

D. Medical professionals

81. When interpreting data, validity and reliability must be taken into consideration. Which of the following is considered the most reliable form of data?

A. Qualitative data

B. Quantitative data

C. Anecdotal information

D. All data is reliable

82. In regard to the definition of medical necessity in insurance contracts, which of the following statements is true?

    A. It is determined by the person reviewing and all decisions are final

    B. It is clear and concise

    C. It is consistent across the industry

    D. They are unclear and open to interpretation

83. Mandatory reporting is required by statutes, which vary state by state. Choose which mandatory reporting is required in all states:

    A. Abuse and Neglect

    B. Medical Neglect

    C. Financial Coercion

    D. Mental Neglect/Cruelty

84. All of the following describe Advance Directives, except:

    A. Are legally executed

    B. Explain the client's healthcare wishes and decisions

    C. Prepared while client is competent

    D. Always involve caregiver input

85. Which source would a case manager use to explore various accommodation options for persons with disabilities in work and educational settings?

    A. Americans with Disabilities Act (ADA) Online Accommodation Calculator

    B. Job Accommodation Network's (JAN) Searchable Online Accommodation Resource (SOAR)

    C. U.S. Department of Labor's Disability Employment Policy

    D. American Civil Liberties Union's (ACLU) Searchable Online Accommodation Resource (SOAR)

86. When dealing with a maladaptive family, the case manager should:

    A. Encourage them to have a single caregiver provide all assistance to the patient so that there is consistency

B. Refer them to support groups or family counseling

C. Close the member to case management as there will be no benefit from the service

D. Arrange for placement of the patient into an appropriate facility

87. Case management is an area of specialty practice within the profession of:

A. Health and Human Services

B. Nursing

C. Social Work

D. Care Coordination

88. Results from this are one of the criteria used to calculate value-based incentive payments in the Hospital Value-Based Purchasing program:

A. The Joint Commission (TJC) survey

B. Cost-benefit analysis reports

C. Hospital Consumer Assessment of Healthcare Providers and Systems (HCAHPS) survey

D. Root cause analysis

89. Which of the following statements regarding experimental treatments is correct?

A. Experimental treatments have little potential for ethical issues

B. The greater good of society as a whole takes precedence over the rights of the individual

C. There must be an equitable system to select who will participate in the experimental treatment

D. A patient does not have to be made aware that the treatment option is experimental as long as all risks are disclosed

90. The case manager demonstrates veracity in all of the following situations except:

A. Speaking on behalf of the client to the insurance company

B. Giving full disclosure about a potential dual relationship

C. Reporting a physician who performs a surgery while intoxicated to the medical board

D. Refusing to lie to the patient regarding his prognosis

91. Which of the following is paid a fixed amount per member per month for contracted healthcare services in a geographical area to a voluntarily enrolled group of people?

    A. PPO

    B. Workers' Compensation

    C. HMO

    D. Managed Care

92. Of the options listed, which is the most desirable for a 60-year-old male following a work-related injury?

    A. To prolong the recovery as long as possible so Social Security and Medicare will take over

    B. To find a different employer to employ him for the same job he had prior to his injury

    C. To return to the same employer in a different job, using transferable skills

    D. To become self-employed

93. After the board-certified case manager fully discloses a conflict of interest to all affected parties, if any objection is made the case manager will:

    A. Seek mediation

    B. Withdraw from further participation in the case

    C. Negotiate an acceptable arrangement for all affected parties

    D. Proceed with case managing the client, the board-certified case manager is only required to disclose the conflict of interest so that all affected parties are aware

94. What is the first step in the negotiation process?

    A. Establish problems and goals

    B. List areas that are agreed upon

    C. Begin work on areas of disagreement

    D. Preparation and understanding the other person's side

95. The type of insurance plan that offers the most flexibility is the:

    A. Point-of-Service Plan (POS)

B. Health Maintenance Origination (HMO)

C. Preferred Provider Organization (PPO)

D. Indemnity Plan

96. A process that uses data mining and specialized software to create statistical models that identifies individuals whose future medical expenses could be significant and would most benefit from appropriate education and intervention through disease management or case management program is known as:

A. Precertification

B. Predictive modeling

C. Health risk assessment

D. Risk stratification

97. A client who is able to effectively communicate and assert his own interests, desires, and needs and is involved in informed decision making is demonstrating:

A. Self-advocacy

B. Informed consent

C. Benevolence

D. Health literacy

98. An insurance program that provides medical benefits and replacement of lost wages for persons suffering from injury or illness that is caused by or occurred in the workplace is:

A. Social Security Disability Insurance (SSDI)

B. Supplemental Security Income (SSI)

C. Workers' Compensation

D. Disability Income Insurance

99. Referral of a client to a healthcare provider who is known to be an unqualified provider is known as:

A. A Medical Error

B. Conflict of Interest

C. A HIPPA Violation

D. Negligent Referral

100. Which of the following is not part of the case management process?

    A. Assess

    B. Report

    C. Coordinate

    D. Evaluate

101. By identifying the percentage of diabetic clients enrolled in case management who have had their HgA1c checked in the last 6 months, the performance improvement team of the case management program is evaluating:

    A. Outcome

    B. Process

    C. Structure

    D. Compliance

102. What best defines an acute illness?

    A. A health condition that requires care from multiple providers

    B. A health condition with a rapid onset and short duration

    C. A health condition that requires ongoing management

    D. A health condition that lasts three months or longer

103. Case manager, Mary, is helping her patient with uncontrolled diabetes improve adherence to their care regimen. What is the first step Mary needs to take?

    A. Mary should get to know and develop a trusting relationship with her patient

    B. Mary should understand the patient's beliefs and attitudes

    C. Mary should understand the patient's level of self-efficacy

    D. Mary should assess the patient's knowledge and understanding of their condition and care regime

104. Which is an example of primary medication non-adherence?

    A. Not taking the prescription

    B. Stopping before completing the course of medication

    C. Not refilling the medication

    D. Not filling the prescription

105. What is a nationally recognized and professionally supported plan of care recommended for the care management of clients with a specific diagnosis or health condition and in a particular care setting?

    A. Standards of care

    B. Evidence-based practice

    C. Care plan

    D. Care guidelines

106. When the case manager is explaining the treatment options available and providing education to the client, the goal is to:

    A. Lead the client to the most cost-efficient treatment plan

    B. Empower the client to be an informed and active decision-maker of his healthcare

    C. Have the client make a decision by the end of the discussion

    D. Encourage the client to obtain a second opinion

107. Which of the following does not provide financial compensation for workers who are unable to work?

    A. Short-term disability insurance (STD)

    B. Social Security Disability Insurance (SSDI)

    C. Family and Medical Leave Act (FMLA)

    D. Workers' Compensation

108. Which of the following is not used by case managers to foster wellness and autonomy?

    A. Advocacy

    B. Education

    C. Coercion

    D. Communication

109. Which Act allows a person extended time off from their job with protection they will not lose their job to care for a family member with a medical condition?

    A. Family Medical Leave Act

    B. Workers' Compensation Act

C. The Health Insurance Portability and Accountability Act

D. American with Disability Act

110. The best interpreter to interpret for a transplant client whose primary language is Italian and speaks "a little English" is:

A. The client's spouse

B. A friend of the client

C. A professional interpreter

D. No interpreter is necessary as the client speaks some English and reading material in Italian can be provided

111. Medication reconciliation is the process of:

A. Educating the patient on how to measure out all their medication

B. Measuring out weekly doses of all medication into a pill container

C. Comparing the patient's medication orders to all the medication a patient is taking

D. Reviewing pharmacy benefits with the patient

112. A healthcare proxy is:

A. A medical document that directs who can make treatment decisions for the client from the date indicated until rescinded

B. A legal document that allows the holder of the document to make treatment decisions for the client

C. A medical document that directs who can make treatment decisions for the client whenever the client is no longer deemed competent to decide for self

D. A legal document that directs who can make treatment decisions for the client whenever the client is no longer deemed competent to decide for self

113. Case managers use the motivational interview to:

A. Motivate and inspire the client to make necessary changes.

B. Help clients to explore and resolve ambivalence.

C. Determine if the client is appropriate for case management.

D. Assess the client's physiological status.

114. Which process is used to identify what, how, and why an adverse event occurred by identifying the factors that contributed to the undesired outcome?

    A. Root Cause Analysis

    B. Critical Pathway

    C. Process Improvement

    D. Internal Investigation

115. Which of the following focuses on the healthcare organization's functions and processes and how these affect the ability to reach desired outcomes and meet the client's needs?

    A. Quality Improvement

    B. Needs and Outcomes Assessment

    C. Outcomes Improvement

    D. Performance Improvement

116. What process best describes the matching of ongoing needs of an individual with the appropriate level and type of care within a setting or across multiple settings?

    A. Transition of Care

    B. Continuum of Care

    C. Coordination of Care

    D. Discharge Planning

117. Which one of the following is used to evaluate an injured worker and assist in determining job placement, job accommodation, or return to work after injury or illness?

    A. Functional capacity evaluation (FCE)

    B. Functional independence measures (FIM)

    C. Instrumental activities of daily living (IADL)

    D. Job analysis

118. All case managers are held to each set of professional standards, excluding:

    A. The Case Management Society of America's Standards of Practice for Case Managers

    B. The Commission for Case Manager Certification Code of Professional Conduct for Case Managers

C. The American Nurses Association Code of Ethics

D. The Case Management Society of America's Code of Ethics for Case Managers

119. A comprehensive set of activities that aims to identify, evaluate, and take corrective action against actual or potential risks that may lead to client or staff injury and result in actual or potential financial or clinical loss, is known as:

A. Risk Management

B. Root Cause Analysis

C. Risk Stratification

D. Risk Mitigation

120. The case manager's role when working with clients with substance abuse is to:

A. Motivate the client to change

B. Support the treatment plan and assist in finding resources

C. Counsel the client

D. Monitor for substance use

121. An array of techniques and methods used for the collection and analysis of data to identify and resolve problems in the system and improve the processes and outcomes of care is known as:

A. Quality Monitoring

B. Outcomes Management

C. Quality Improvement

D. Outcomes Improvement

122. Which statement about Medicare Hospice benefit is correct?

A. Given in benefit periods of 90 days each for the first and second periods

B. Hospice providers can be changed multiple times during a benefit period

C. Hospice is not a covered benefit under Medicare

D. A patient can keep the normal Medicare hospital benefit

123. The Social Determinants of Health can have a major impact on the ability of the client to reach optimum health and wellness. Assessing for the Social Determinants of Health may include:

A. Access to healthcare services, exposure to toxic substances, and genetic factors

B. Access to transportation, economic stability, and gender

C. Gender, access to educational, economic, and job opportunities

D. Availability of community-based resources in support of community living and opportunities for recreational and leisure-time activities

124. The case manager and treating physician have informed the client of the options available, including the risks and benefits of each option, and answered the client's questions. By respecting the client's decision they are demonstrating which of the five ethical principles?

A. Non-malfeasance

B. Autonomy

C. Fidelity

D. Justice

125. Case Management is what type of process?

A. Independent

B. Organizational

C. Collaborative

D. Educational

126. Standards of care are:

A. Statements that delineate care that is expected to be provided to all clients based on the best scientific knowledge, current outcomes data, and clinical expertise

B. Statements of an acceptable level of performance or expectation for professional intervention or behavior associated with one's professional practice

C. Statements that delineate care that is expected to be provided to most clients based on the best scientific knowledge, current outcomes data, and clinical expertise

D. Only of relevance to physicians and therefore not relevant to case management

127. Amy is a 68-year-old woman who was living alone independently prior to a prolonged hospitalization for septicemia. She currently is medically stable but is unable to safely ambulate without assistance or navigate the stairs to get to her 2nd-floor bathroom. She is able to tolerate at least 3 hours of therapy a day. The most appropriate rehabilitation setting for her post-hospitalization is:

A. Home health

B. Outpatient rehabilitation

C. She will need to remain in the acute care hospital until she can safely return home

D. Inpatient rehabilitation

128. Psychological and neuropsychological assessments can be important to creating an appropriate case management plan. Which of the following is not an assessment tool for psychological and neuropsychological status?

A. DSM-IV

B. Glasgow Coma Score (GCS)

C. Motivational Interviewing (MI)

D. Minnesota Multiphasic Personality Inventory (MMPI)

129. A health coach is working with a client on weight loss. What is the most important thing the health coach should do when setting goals?

A. Set small, achievable goals for the client

B. Set a long-term goal for the client to have a normal BMI

C. Not make the client aware of the goal, so that they do not feel pressured

D. Assist the client to set goals that are meaningful to the client

130. Medical Necessity is:

A. A service or treatment ordered by an in-network physician

B. Needed to diagnose and treat a medical condition as per recognized standards

C. A service or treatment provided under the patient's insurance contract

D. A service identified in the proposed plan of care

131. Which of the following is an example of a hard cost saving as a result of case management?

A. Otherwise medically stable patient is sent home with daily visits to an outpatient clinic for his daily dose of IV antibiotic

B. Avoidance of 30-day hospital readmission

C. Prevention of medical complications from misuse of medication

D. Avoidance of emergency department visits after the case manager assists the client in finding a primary care physician

132. In regard to the psychosocial aspects of chronic illness and disability, it is important for the case manager to know:

A. All patients with a catastrophic illness or injury will suffer from depression and should be placed on antidepressant medication prophylactically

B. All patients who suffer a spinal cord injury will have similar psychological responses

C. A primary goal is to help the client realize they will never again be a productive member of society and encourage them to apply for social security disability insurance

D. The more self-efficacy a client has, the more likely he or she will persevere when obstacles arise

133. If the case manager discovers that the client's cultural beliefs are very different from the case manager's, the case manager should:

A. Respect the client's beliefs, even though she may not agree with them

B. Close the client to case management

C. Transfer the client's case to another case manager with similar cultural beliefs

D. Confront the client, informing them that their beliefs are incorrect

134. When screening for patients to consider for case management services, which one is not appropriate?

A. 52-year-old female with renal cell carcinoma

B. 88-year-old male who resides in a skilled nursing facility and developed a urinary tract infection

C. 49-year-old male with 6 ER visits and 2 inpatient hospitalizations in the last 2 months

D. 25-year-old female post motor vehicle accident who sustained pelvic and bilateral lower extremity fractures and has no family or support system

135. Which of the following would be used to measure a 6-year-old's level of functional independence following a motor vehicle accident?

A. Functional Independence Measure (FIM)

B. Functional Capacity Assessment (FCA)

C. Instrumental Activities of Daily Living (IADL) assessment

D. WeeFIM

136. Sue is a 25-year-old client with aggressive breast cancer. During your initial assessment, she identified as being a devout Catholic. During your last interactions, she stated she, "does not know why God is punishing her like this. She has always been a good Catholic." Which of the following would be the best to refer Sue to?

A. A support group for breast cancer patients

B. A counselor

C. A psychiatrist

D. A priest

137. The set of standards identified by the Centers for Medicare and Medicaid Services (CMS) based on scientific evidence of improved patient outcomes to hospitalized patients, which have been endorsed by both government and commercial payers, are known as:

A. Minimum Data Set

B. Standards of Care

C. Conditions of Participation

D. Core Measures

138. Which of the following takes place prior to services being rendered to determine if the requested service is medically necessary?

A. Concurrent review

B. Precertification

C. Retrospective review

D. Review for referral to case management

139. A tool case managers can use to assess for substance abuse or addiction is:

A. CAGE Tool

B. Glasgow Coma Scale

C. The Mini-Mental Exam

D. Hamilton D

140. When must an individual decide to elect COBRA?

    A. Within 90 days of termination of plan coverage

    B. Before leaving the covered employment

    C. Within 60 days of termination of plan coverage

    D. The individual has up to 6 months to decide

141. The use of information and knowledge gained from outcomes monitoring to achieve optimal client outcomes through improved clinical decision making and service delivery is known as:

    A. Outcome indicators

    B. Outcome management

    C. Outcome measurement

    D. Outcome optimization

142. Asking the client questions such as "Are you confident filling out medical forms by yourself?" and "How well do you understand your medical conditions?" are ways that the case manager assesses for:

    A. Health literacy

    B. Illiteracy

    C. Compliance with the plan of care

    D. Language barriers

143. Which criteria must be met to be eligible for hospice?

    A. A signed DNR

    B. A physician certifies that the patient has a life expectancy of 6 months or less

    C. Intractable pain

    D. The need for palliative care

144. A nationally standardized survey of patients' perspectives of their hospital experience developed by Centers for Medicare and Medicaid Services (CMS) which allows for an objective comparison of hospitals on topics that are important to consumers is:

    A. CMS Hospital Experience Survey

B. Hospital Consumer Assessment of Healthcare Providers and Systems (HCAHPS)

C. The Joint Commission (TJC) Survey

D. Patient Perspective Survey (PPS)

145. A caregiver is keeping a client with dementia sedated to the point that they sleep most of the day. This is:

A. Neglect

B. Physical abuse

C. Psychological abuse

D. An acceptable safety measure

146. Which of the following is false regarding the coordination of benefits (COB)?

A. COB prevents duplicate payment for services

B. COB is mandated by the federal government

C. Following COB guidelines is voluntary

D. COB determines which policy pays primary when an individual is covered by more than one insurance policy

147. An extended or severe illness will require modifications of family responsibilities. Adaptive families:

A. Rely on a single person to provide all assistance to the patient

B. Deny the patient's condition

C. Foster patient dependency

D. Seek and accept help

148. The main purpose of a concurrent review of a hospitalized patient is to:

A. Assess the need for continued hospitalization

B. Assess for discharge planning needs

C. Determine medical necessity for admission

D. Screen for the need for case management

149. A process used to identify the basic or causal factors that contribute to the occurrence of a sentinel event is:

A. Root cause analysis

B. Risk management

C. Sentinel event investigation

D. Quality management

150. Mr. Kim tells you that his sister brings him "herbs and teas" to help fight his cancer. He states he did not tell his doctor, as he didn't think it was important. You should instruct Mr. Kim to:

A. Give his doctor the names of any herbs and teas he is taking as they may interact with his other medications.

B. Continue taking these herbs and teas, if he believes they are working it may provide a placebo effect.

C. Stop taking the herbs and teas immediately.

D. Check with his pharmacist to see if these teas and herbs are safe to take.

Practice Test Answer Key

1. Answer: C

   Rationale: The social determinants of health impact the ability to carry out the plan of care and are therefore important to case managers. They can affect all socioeconomic levels. Age, race, and gender are genetic factors and are not included in the social determinants of health.

2. Answer: D

   Rationale: Screening and assessment tools are used by case managers and other settings to classify clients into low, moderate, or high-risk categories. Answers A, B, and C are additional steps in the case management process.

3. Answer: C

   Rationale: Board-certified case managers may not participate in unprofessional behavior, such as disclosing information about a client via social media.

4. Answer: C

   Rationale: A cost-benefit report can be used to formally document monetary savings related to case management involvement including hard and soft cost savings, as well as justify a more costly intervention. Quality improvement reports have the purpose of demonstrating quality.

5. Answers: B

   Rationale: The remainder are examples of maladaptive family behaviors.

6. Answer: A

   Rationale: Hard Savings are directly related to the case manager's actions. The other choices are examples of soft savings. Soft savings are potential savings and are difficult to measure.

7. Answer: B

   Rationale: CCMC in their Glossary of Terms defines Permanent Partial Disability as a disability that is caused by either a work-related injury or an occupational illness resulting in some form of permanent impairment that makes a worker unable to perform at their full capacity. An example is the loss of vision in one eye or amputation of a finger on one hand (CCMC, 2019).

8. Answer: D

   Rationale: CCMC in its Glossary of Terms defines the functional capacity evaluation as a systematic process of assessing an individual's physical capacities and functional abilities. The FCE matches human performance levels to the demands of a specific job, work activity, or occupation. It establishes the physical level of work an individual can perform (CCMC, 2019).

9. Answer: B

Rationale: Each response may occur when clients are receiving treatment, but only b describes an underpinning of patient rights.

10. Answer: B

Rationale: This patient has a $250 deductible and a co-pay of $25 per visit. At the time of the visit, she has satisfied $200 of her deductible and has $50 left. The charge for the visit is $400. The patient is responsible for the remaining $50 and the co-pay of $25.

11. Answer: B

Rationale: Dual Diagnosis refers to clients with coexisting mental illness and substance abuse disorders. The mental illness must meet the criteria for diagnosis by the Diagnostic and Statistical Manual of Mental Disorders (DSM-5).

12. Answer: B

Rationale: CCMC in its Glossary of Terms defines work hardening as a program that focuses on work endurance and uses real or simulated job tasks and duties and progressively graded conditioning exercises based on the worker's measured tolerance to ultimately return the worker to gainful employment (CCMC, 2019).

13. Answer: D

Rationale: Although job discrimination may indirectly affect access to healthcare due to lack of employer insurance, answers A, B, and C are better answers.

14. Answer: B

Rationale: Accreditation is not mandatory and usually requires more than a minimum standard of quality to be met.

15. Answer: B

Rationale: The living will is a legal document that directs the healthcare provider in holding or withdrawing life support measures. It is usually prepared by the patient while he is competent, indicating the patient's wishes.

16. Answer: A

Rationale: The definition for Employability is having the skills and training that are commonly necessary in the labor market to be gainfully employed on a reasonably continuous basis, when considering the person's age, education, experience, physical, and mental capacities due to industrial injury or disease (CCMC, 2019).

17. Answer: B

Rationale: Case managers that are required to prepare patient reports should always prepare a report at case closure as this is the only report that will show the complete case and will serve as an update to any previous reports.

18. Answer: C

Rationale: CMSA lists these as the five basic ethical principles for case managers (CMSA, 2016).

19. Answer: A

Rationale: In the contemplation phase, a client is considering a change but is not ready to commit.

20. Answer: A

Rationale: Workers' compensation laws were developed in 1908 by federal statute, but they are enforced on the state level. Workers' compensation varies from state to state.

21. Answer: C

Rationale: Although assessing for barriers to compliance with the care plan is an important task for the case manager to complete, it does not foster or encourage self-efficacy in the client. Self-efficacy is one's belief in his or her own ability to succeed. The case manager can foster and encourage self-efficacy in the client by providing affirmation, motivation, and encouragement. She can facilitate goal setting that will promote mastery by helping the client create small, attainable goals. The case manager can also assist the client reach optimal physical and psychological function by making referrals as needed.

22. Answer: C

Rationale: Job accommodation is defined as a reasonable adjustment to a job or work environment that makes it possible for an individual with a disability to perform job duties. Accommodations may include specialized equipment, facility modifications, adjustments to work schedules or job duties, as well as a whole range of other creative solutions (United States Department of Labor, 2010).

23. Answer: C

Rationale: Incident Reports document potential and actual risks.

24. Answer: A

Rationale: Developing an individualized case management plan is the main objective during the planning step. Answers: b, c, d, Patient goals can then be formulated through gathering information from the patient and caregiver.

25. Answer: B

Rationale: The Americans with Disabilities Act prohibits workplace discrimination against individuals with, or with a history of, psychiatric disabilities not controlled by medication. It does not, however, protect criminal diagnoses, such as pyromania or kleptomania.

26. Answer: D

Rationale: Spiritual practices tend to improve coping skills, provide optimism and hope, promote healthy behavior, decrease feelings of depression and anxiety, and encourage a sense of relaxation. By relieving stressful feelings and promoting healthy ones, spirituality can positively influence immune, cardiovascular, hormonal, and nervous systems.

27. Answer: B

Rationale: The Ticket To Work Program is in place to give those 18-64 who are collecting Social Security Disability a way to test if they can return to a paid job without losing their Disability payments.

28. Answer: A

Rationale: Of the options listed, only the job analysis is used to identify and determine the job duties and requirements for a given job.

29. Answer: D

Rationale: All of the answers are examples of healthcare analytic tools that can be used to identify at-risk individuals who may benefit from case management services except for the Case Management Survey. The Case management survey assesses the client's satisfaction with case management services.

30. Answer: B

Rationale: A benefit period begins when first admitted to the hospital. It ends when the patient has been out of the hospital or an SNF for at least 60 days. This patient returned after one month or 30 days. If the patient stays in the hospital or transfers to an SNF, a copay will be required beginning on day 61 of the benefit period and continues through day 90.

31. Answer: A

   Rationale: The engaged client will be taking action, such as exercising regularly, taking medications as prescribed, or monitoring blood sugars.

32. Answer: D

   Rationale: Undue hardship can refer to accommodations that cause financial difficulty, are disruptive to the workplace, or fundamentally change the operation of the business.

33. Answer: A

   Rationale: CCMC in its Glossary of Terms defines the claims adjuster as; an insurance professional who investigates claims by interviewing the claimant and other involved parties (e.g., Employers and witnesses), reviews related records to determine the degree of liability and damages and assures that an insurance policy exists and covers the claimed damages. In healthcare, a claims adjuster also assures that medical care is available to the worker as needed based on the injury or occupational illness (CCMC, 2019).

34. Answer: A

   Rationale: Managed Care: A system of healthcare delivery that aims to provide a generalized structure and focus when managing the use, access, cost, quality, and effectiveness of healthcare services. Links the patient to provider services. PPOs, EPOs, and HMOs are types of managed care.

35. Answer: B

   Rationale: Fraud is defined as an intentional deception or misrepresentation that someone makes, knowing it is false, that could result in an unauthorized payment (CCMC, 2019).

36. Answer: C

   Rational: CCMC in their Glossary of Terms states the cost-benefit analysis is a technique or systematic process used to calculate and compare the benefits and cost of an action, intervention, service, or treatment, and to determine how well, or how poorly, it will turn out. This analysis reveals whether the benefits outweigh the cost, and by how much so that the involved party is able to make the appropriate decision(s) (CCMC, 2017).

37. Answer: D

   Rationale: "D" is not a Conflict Resolution strategy. They include collaboration, negotiation, accommodation, competitive, and avoidance.

38. Answer: C

Rationale: Instrumental Activities of Daily Living (IADL) tool assesses:
- Ability to use the telephone
- Shopping
- Food Preparation
- Housekeeping
- Laundry
- Mode of Transportation
- Responsibility for own Medications
- Ability to handle finances

39. Answer: B

Rationale: After a work-related injury, the goal is for the worker to achieve maximum medical improvement and return to work as soon as possible. The case manager may coordinate care and perform other duties, but those duties are not the goal.

40. Answer: B

Rational: CCMC in its Glossary of Terms defines a quality indicator as a predetermined measure for assessing quality; a metric (CCMC, 2019).

41. Answer: C

Rationale: According to The American Psychiatric Association's Diagnostic and Statistical Manual of Mental Disorders, 5th Edition (DSM-5), substance abuse is a maladaptive pattern of substance use leading to clinically significant impairment or distress.

42. Answer: A

Rationale: Case managers are not to make decisions for their clients, but rather to educate their clients based on the best evidence available.

43. Answer: A

Rationale: Measures of structure include the environment of care and practice that have a direct or indirect impact on outcomes of care. Percentage of clients screened for breast cancer is a measure of process.

44. Answer: C

Rationale: The ADA protects prospective applicants from being asked about their medical history or status.

45. Answer: A

Rationale: It is important to conduct a comprehensive assessment with the client to identify problems, care needs, and interests. Others are helpful, but the primary source of information should be the client.

46. Answer: D

Rationale: A and B are not ethical principles. Non-maleficence is doing no harm. By working with the QA team to improve outcomes, the case manager is helping to ensure harm is not done.

47. Answer: C

Rationale: Spirituality is a broad concept with many perspectives. In general, it includes a sense of connection to something bigger than ourselves. For some people, spirituality is synonymous with religion, but a person does not have to have a religious belief to be spiritual. It is important for the case manager to have an understanding of clients' spiritual and religious views, as the views often impact choices they make in regard to healthcare.

48. Answer: D

Rationale: A life care plan provides an organized, concise plan for current and future needs for individuals who have experienced catastrophic injury or have chronic health care needs.

49. Answer: C

Rationale: Managed care is a system of healthcare delivery whose goal is to maintain quality, cost-effective care by managing the use, access, cost, quality, and effectiveness of services.

50. Answer: B

Rationale: The Newest Vital Sign – A tool that tests literacy skills for both numbers and words.

51. Answer: D

Rationale: The evaluation step of the case management process focuses on the effectiveness of the plan of care and its effect on the client's condition. Evaluating outcomes looks at many aspects such as financial evaluation, clinical outcomes self-care management ability, knowledge of health conditions, and plan of care.

52. Answer: A

Rationale: The assessment is self-administered therefore it is not time-consuming for the case manager to administer.

53. Answer: C

Rationale: Emotional/psychological abuse is inflicting anguish, pain or distress through verbal or nonverbal acts resulting in trauma. Some examples include verbal assaults, insults, threats, coercion, and Intimidation.

54. Answer: A

Rationale: To provide prescription medication in the most cost-effective manner.

55. Answer: B

Rationale: 5 Stages of Change

1. In the pre-contemplation stage, the individual does not intend to take action in the foreseeable future.

2. In the contemplation stage, the individual considers a change in the next six months but has not committed to it. He may be open to information on the benefits of change and how to successfully do so.

3. In the preparation stage, the client actively plans to make changes within the next month and may have taken small steps toward change.

4. Action is the stage when the individual has successfully made a change and has sustained it for less than six months.

5. When the individual has sustained the change for more than 6 months, maintenance has been achieved.

56. Answer: D

Rationale: Detoxification alone does not address the psychological, social, and behavioral problems associated with addiction and therefore does not typically produce lasting behavioral change necessary for recovery. Therefore, it should be followed by ongoing drug addiction treatment.

57. Answer: D

Rationale: The role of an advocate speaks on behalf of another person and promotes their cause.

58. Answer: A

Rationale: Medicare Part A covers hospice services. It only covers prescriptions that are related to the hospice diagnosis and has 2 benefit periods of 90 days each followed by unlimited 60 day periods. There is no deductible for hospice care.

59. Answer: A

Rationale: "A" is correct; no other organization listed is as broad scope as an Area Agency on Aging which is a clearinghouse for many different programs and organizations.

60. Answer: D

Rationale: Workers' compensation case managers focus on vocational activities and collaborate with the employer to facilitate returning the employee to gainful employment.

61. Answer: D

Rationale: Although the other accreditations may be helpful, the best answer for a rehabilitation facility is CARF as it is a private, nonprofit organization that establishes standards of quality for services to people with disabilities and offers voluntary accreditation for rehabilitation facilities based on a set of nationally recognized standards (CCMC, 2017).

62. Answer: C

Rationale: Homecare services are covered for homebound patients that require skilled services provided by a licensed professional. Assistance with ADLs is custodial care. Custodial care is not covered by Medicare.

63. Answer: A

Rationale: The MMPI is a psychological test that assesses personality traits and psychopathology. It is most commonly used by mental health professionals to assess and diagnose mental illness. It can only be given and interpreted by a psychologist trained to do so.

64. Answer: C

Rationale: Under COB rules, the insurance plan covering the individual as an employee is the primary payer.

65. Answer: D

Rationale: Goals and objectives of case management include achieving optimal outcomes, quality of care, appropriate use of services and resources, optimum health, and functioning for the client.

66. Answer: D

Rationale: SSDI is an earned benefit provided to disabled workers between the ages of 18 and 65. When the individual turns 65, they become eligible for traditional Social Security.

67. Answer: A

Rationale: CCMC in its Glossary of Terms states that benchmarking is an act of comparing a work process with that of the best competitor. Through this process, one is able to identify what performance measure levels must be surpassed. Benchmarking assists an organization in assessing its strengths and weaknesses and in finding and implementing best practices (CCMC, 2017).

68. Answer: A

Rationale: The Americans with Disabilities Act, or ADA, defines an individual with a disability as a person who: 1) has a physical or mental impairment that substantially limits a major life activity, 2) has a record or history of a substantially limiting impairment, or 3) is regarded or perceived by an employer as having a substantially limiting impairment.

69. Answer: B

Rationale: Risk factors for low health literacy include:

• Older adults

• Racial and ethnic minorities

• Those having less than a high school degree or GED

• Individuals whose income is at or below the poverty level

• Non-native speakers of English

70. Answer: B

Rationale: Answers, a, c, and d present conflicts of interest between the case manager and multiple employers that conflict with each other, and potentially impede the ability of the case manager to engage in one role objectively vs. the other.

71. Answer: D

Rationale: The Americans with Disabilities Act provides protection for qualified applicants and employees with drug addiction if they have been successfully rehabilitated and no longer use drugs or alcohol. It does not protect employees who are currently using drugs or alcohol.

72. Answer: B

Rationale: Case management is a collaborative process that assesses, plans, implements, coordinates, monitors, and evaluates the options and services required to meet the client's health and human service needs. It is characterized by advocacy, communication, and resource management and promotes quality and cost-effective interventions and outcomes.

73. Answer: A

Rationale: Self-efficacy is one's belief in his or her own ability to succeed, and it plays a major role in the client's outcome. The more self-efficacy a client possesses, the more likely he or she will persevere when obstacles arise.

74. Answer: D

Rationale: Performance improvement can be prospective or retrospective, and aims to improve how things are done. There are several measurements for performance improvement, including process, structure, and outcomes.

75. Answer: A

Rationale: To qualify for hospice under Medicare Part A, a physician must certify that the patient has a life expectancy of 6 months or less. The patient must also waive normal Medicare hospital benefits and not pursue further curative treatment. That includes clinical trials at any phase.

76. Answer: B

Rationale: Two types of negotiation are: Aggressive or hardball, which aims to result in a winner and a loser, and cooperative negotiation seeks a win-win outcome and results in the best for everyone.

77. Answer D

Rationale: CCMC in their Glossary of Terms defines quality assurance as the use of activities and programs to ensure the quality of patient care. These activities and programs are designed to monitor, prevent, and correct quality deficiencies and noncompliance with the standards of care and practice (CCMC, 2017).

78. Answer: C

Rationale: PSDA amends Title XVIII- (Medicare) and Title XIX (Medicaid) requiring all inpatient facilities, Home Health agencies, hospice programs and managed care companies to recognize these documents.

79. Answer: C

Rationale: Workers' compensation pays for medical care for work-related injuries beginning immediately after the injury occurs.

80. Answer: A

Rationale: Health coaching is secondary prevention. Clients who already have a chronic disease can benefit from learning to manage the disease.

81. Answer: B

Rationale: Quantitative data is considered the most reliable as it has the least room for interpretation or bias.

82. Answer: D

Rationale: Health insurance contracts usually define medical necessity as care that is appropriate, reasonable, and necessary. Unfortunately, these are subjective terms and determination of medical necessity can vary based on the interpretation of these terms.

83. Answer: A

Rationale: Most healthcare professionals are mandatory reporters of abuse and neglect.

84. Answer: D

Rationale: Caregivers are not always involved in Advanced Directives (CCMC, 2019).

85. Answer: B

Rationale: JAN represents the most comprehensive resource for job accommodations available.

86. Answer: B

Rationale: The case manager can make a referral to family counseling or support groups. She can also encourage the family to maintain as much of their normal routine as possible.

87. Answer: A

Rationale: According to CCMC's website, Case management is an area of specialty practice within one's health and human services profession.

88. Answer: C

Rationale: The Affordable Care Act includes the Hospital Consumer Assessment of Healthcare Providers and Systems (HCAHPS) data among the measures used to calculate value-based incentive payments in the Hospital Value-Based Purchasing program.

89. Answer: C

Rationale: It is unethical to give preference when deciding who will be permitted to participate in experimental treatment.

90. Answer: A

Rationale: "Veracity is the legal principle that states that a health professional should be honest and give full disclosure; abstain from misrepresentation or deceit; report known lapses of the standards of care to the proper agencies. (Mosby's Dental Dictionary, 2nd Ed. 2008)" (CCMC, 2019). Advocacy is speaking on behalf of the client.

91. Answer: C

Rationale: Health Maintenance Organization (HMO): An organization that provides or arranges for coverage of designated health services needed by plan members for a fixed prepaid premium. There are four basic models of HMOs: group model, individual practice association (IPA), network model, and staff model. Under the Federal HMO Act, an organization must possess the following to call itself an HMO: (1) an organized system for providing healthcare in a geographical area, (2) an agreed-on set of basic and supplemental health maintenance and treatment services, and (3) a voluntarily enrolled group of people (CCMC, 2017).

92. Answer: C

Rationale: After a work-related injury, the goal is for the worker to achieve maximum medical improvement and to return to work as soon as possible. The return to work options are evaluated in the following order:

1. Same job, same employer

2. Modified job, same employer

3. Different job, same employer, using transferable skills

4. Same job, different employer

5. Different job, different employer, using transferable skills

6. Training for different job with same or different employer

7. Self-employment

93. Answer: B

Rationale: Any conflict of interest must be fully disclosed to all affected parties, and if any objection is made, the board-certified case manager will withdraw from further participation in the case (CCMC Code of Professional Conduct for Case Managers, 2017).

94. Answer: D

Rationale: Negotiation processes first start with understanding the other person's side before the meeting. Establishing problems and goals, listing areas that are agreed upon, and working on areas of disagreement are the following steps.

95. Answer: D

Rationale: Indemnity plans offer the most flexibility because they do not have restrictions on which provider the insured can use. Indemnity benefits usually pay after the provider has billed the patient, and the insured person is reimbursed by the company. Also, know as fee-for-service where providers are paid for each service performed, as opposed to capitation.

96. Answer: B

Rationale: Predictive modeling is a process used in data mining, usually automated, and employs specialized software applications to create a statistical model of future behavior that forecasts probabilities and trends. Case management programs can use this information to identify individuals whose future medical expenses could be significant and would most benefit from appropriate education and intervention through disease management or case management program.

Risk stratification assigns a level of risk (low, moderate, high) based on a set of predetermined criteria using health assessments and biomedical screening tools.

97. Answer: A

Rationale: Self-advocacy is effectively communicating and asserting one's own interests, desires, and needs.

98. Answer: C

Rationale: An insurance program that provides medical benefits and replacement of lost wages for persons suffering from injury or illness that is caused by or occurred in the workplace. It is an insurance system for industrial and work injury, regulated primarily among the separate states, but regulated in certain specified occupations by the federal government (CCMC, 2019).

99. Answer: D

Rationale: Negligent referral is defined as referring a client to a healthcare provider who is unqualified.

100. Answer B

Rationale: Although case managers may complete reports, and report to others, this is not part of the case management process.

101. Answer: B

Rationale: Measures of process examine what is actually done in giving and receiving care and how well clinical guidelines are followed. For example, the percentage of clients screened for colon cancer.

Outcome is incorrect because it measures the health status of the patient as a result of healthcare. For example the number of diabetics with acceptable HgA1c levels.

Compliance is incorrect as we do not know if the clients were offered the test.

102. Answer: B

Rationale: Acute diseases are characterized by rapid onset with a short duration, where chronic diseases require ongoing management of a health condition or disease that lasts three months or longer.

103. Answer: D

Rationale: The first step in helping a client is to understand the patient's knowledge of their condition. Developing a trusting relationship, understanding their beliefs, attitudes and self-efficacy are all ways a case manager can help increase a client's adherence.

104. Answer: D

Rationale: Nonadherence to medications can be primary or secondary reasons. Primary nonadherence takes the form of not filling the prescription.

105. Answer: D

Rationale: CCMC in its Glossary of Terms defines care guidelines as a nationally recognized and professionally supported plan of care recommended for the care management of clients with a specific diagnosis or health condition and in a particular care setting (CCMC, 2017).

106. Answer: B

Rationale: Case managers empower patients to be informed and active decision-makers in their healthcare by explaining treatment options available and providing education on disease or injury, community resources, and insurance coverage. The case manager is never to make a decision for the client but guides the client in the decision making process.

107. Answer: C

Rationale: The FMLA entitles eligible employees of covered employers to take unpaid, job-protected leave for specified family and medical reasons with continuation of group health insurance coverage under the same terms and conditions as if the employee had not taken leave.

108. Answer: C

Rationale: CCMC's Philosophy of Case Management states case management facilitates the achievement of client wellness and autonomy through advocacy, assessment, planning, communication, education, resource management, and service facilitation.

109. Answer: A

Rationale: The Family Medical Leave Act allows people to take an extended period of time due to an illness or to care for a family member with protection that they will have a job when they return. The FMLA is not a source of income but does protect the employee's job.

110. Answer: C

Rationale: Although friends and family may be a convenient source of interpretation, they should not be the primary interpreter. The client may not feel comfortable disclosing some information to family members or friends regarding their private health matters. The ability of the client to speak "a little" English does not ensure he is properly understanding the information provided.

111. Answer: C

Rationale: Medication reconciliation is the process of comparing a patient's medication orders to all the medications that the patient has been taking (JCAHO).

112. Answer: D

Rationale: CCMC defines a healthcare proxy as, "a legal document that directs the healthcare provider/agency in whom to contact for approval/consent of treatment decisions or options whenever the client is no longer deemed competent to decide for self" (CCMC, 2019).

113. Answer: B

Rationale: The motivational interview is a method that works on facilitating and engaging intrinsic motivation within the client in order to change behavior. The motivational interview is a goal-oriented, client-centered counseling style for eliciting behavior change by helping clients to explore and resolve ambivalence.

114. Answer: A

Rationale: A Root Cause Analysis is a process used by healthcare providers and administrators to identify the basic or causal factors that contribute to variation in performance and outcomes or underlie the occurrence of a sentinel event (CCMC, 2019).

115. Answer: D

Rationale: CCMC in their Glossary of Terms defines performance improvement as the continuous study and adaption of the functions and processes of a healthcare organization to increase the probability of achieving desired outcomes and to better meet the needs of the clients (CCMC, 2017).

116. Answer: B

Rationale: The continuum of care matches ongoing needs of the individuals with the appropriate level of care and type of health, medical, financial, legal, and psychosocial services within a setting or across multiple settings.

117. Answer: A

Rationale: Functional Capacity Evaluation (FCE): A systematic process of assessing an individual's physical capacities and functional abilities. The FCE matches human performance levels to the demands of a specific job or work activity or occupation. It establishes the physical level of work an individual can perform. The FCE is useful in determining job placement, job accommodation, or return to work after injury or illness. FCEs can provide objective information regarding functional workability in the determination of occupational disability status (CCMC, 2019).

118. Answer: C

Rationale: Not all case managers are nurses, so they are not held to the Standards of the American Nurses Association Code of Ethics.

119. Answer: A

Rationale: Risk management is defined by CCMC in its Glossary of Terms as, the science of the identification, evaluation, and treatment of actual or potential financial or clinical losses. Usually occurs through a formal program that attempts to avoid, prevent, or minimize negative results. The program consists of a comprehensive set of activities that aims to identify, evaluate, and take corrective action against risks that may lead to client or staff injury with resulting financial loss or legal liability (CCMC, 2019).

120. Answer: B

Rationale: The case manager's role is to support the treatment plan, provide encouragement to the patient, and assist them in finding available resources. Clients with substance abuse often have dual diagnosis and need treatment for coexisting mental illness.

121. Answer: C

Rationale: CCMC in its Glossary of Terms defines quality improvement as an array of techniques and methods used for the collection and analysis of data gathered in the course of current healthcare practice in a defined care setting, to identify and resolve problems in the system and improve the processes and outcomes of care (CCMC, 2017).

122. Answer: A

Rationale: Hospice under Medicare is given in benefit periods of 90 days each for the first and second periods. The following periods are 60 days and are unlimited.

123. Answer: D

Rationale: Genetic factors, age, and gender are fixed and are not included in the social determinants of health. Examples of social determinants include:

- Availability of resources to meet daily needs (e.g., safe housing and local food markets)
- Access to educational, economic, and job opportunities
- Access to health care services
- Availability of community-based resources in support of community living and opportunities for recreational and leisure-time activities
- Transportation options
- Social support
- Language/Literacy
- Access to mass media and emerging technologies (e.g., cell phones, the Internet, and social media)
- Exposure to toxic substances and other hazards
- Built environment, such as buildings, sidewalks, bike lanes, and roads

124. Answer: B

Rationale: Autonomy is the ethical principle that respects the individual's rights to make their own decisions and to self-determine a course of action.

125. Answer: C

Rationale: Case management is a collaborative process that assesses, plans, implements, coordinates, monitors, and evaluates the options and services required to meet the client's health and human service needs. It is characterized by advocacy, communication, and resource management, and promotes quality and cost-effective interventions and outcomes.

126. Answer: A

Rationale: CCMC in its Glossary of Terms defines standards of care as statements that delineate care that is expected to be provided to all clients. They include predefined outcomes of care clients can expect from providers and are accepted within the community of professionals, based upon the best scientific knowledge, current outcomes data, and clinical expertise (CCMC, 2017). Answer B is the definition of standards of practice.

127. Answer: D

Rationale: A and B are incorrect because she can not safely return home. C is incorrect as she is medically stable and no longer requires acute level of care.

128. Answer: C

Rationale: Motivational Interviewing is an interview technique that focuses on helping the client discover his or her motivation for change.

129. Answer: D

Rationale: During the motivational interview, the health coach helps the client discover issues that are most concerning to the client and discovers the inner motivations to make necessary changes. This information can then be used to make goals that are meaningful to the client, increasing the likelihood of successfully achieving the goals. The health coach should not make goals for the client, but should assist the client in setting goals.

130. Answer: B

Rationale: Medically necessary services are those needed to diagnose and treat a medical condition in accordance with nationally recognized standards.

131. Answer: A

Rationale: A is the only answer that provides an example of hard saving that a case manager can claim. The others are examples of soft savings.

132. Answer: D

Rationale: Not all patients will be affected in the same way by a chronic or catastrophic illness. How an individual is affected may be influenced by numerous factors. Self-efficacy is one's belief in his or her own ability to succeed. The more self-efficacy a client possesses, the more likely he or she will persevere when obstacles arise.

133. Answer: A

Rationale: The client's cultural beliefs may be very different from the case manager's. This can influence how a case manager views her client. The case manager must respect the client's beliefs, even though she may not agree with them. It can be helpful to acknowledge the cultural differences with the client and reassure the client that the case manager's job is to educate him and support his decisions.

134. Answer: B

Rationale: The case manager will have little impact on a resident of a skilled nursing facility who should have a team of providers.

135. Answer: D

Rationale: The WeeFIM is used to measure functional independence in children.

136. Answer: D

Rationale: Although Sue may benefit from any of these services, her primary struggle is spiritual. Because of her devout faith, a priest would be the most appropriate initial referral.

137. Answer: D

Rationale: Core Measures are standards that have been shown through scientific evidence to improve patient outcomes, and they set the standard for care provided to patients while in the hospital.

The Core Quality Measures Collaborative established agreed-upon core measure sets that are coordinated across both government and commercial payers.

138. Answer: B

Rationale: Precertification is the process of obtaining and documenting advanced approval from the health plan by the provider before delivering the medical services needed. This is required when services are of a non-emergent nature (CCMC, 2017).

139. Answer: A

Rationale: CAGE is an assessment tool used to screen for substance abuse.

140. Answer: C

Rationale: An individual must elect within 60 days of termination of plan coverage.

141. Answer: B

Rationale: CCMC in their Glossary of Terms defines outcomes management as the use of information and knowledge gained from outcomes monitoring to achieve optimal client outcomes through improved clinical decision making and service delivery (CCMC, 2017). Answer A, Outcome indicators, are metrics used to examine and evaluate the results of the care delivered. Answer B, outcomes measurement, is the systematic, quantitative observation, at a point in time, of outcome indicators (CCMC, 2017).

142. Answer: A

Rationale: Health literacy is the ability to obtain, communicate, process, and understand basic health information. Signs that a patient may have low health literacy include making statements that another family member handles their medications, or deferring questions about their health history to a family member.

143. Answer: B

Rationale: The primary criteria for hospice is certification from a physician of a life expectancy of 6 months or less. Although a signed DNR is preferred, it is not required in all hospice programs to initiate hospice care. Treatment for intractable pain and palliative care can be provided by a hospice program, but can also be provided by other healthcare providers in the absence of a terminal diagnosis.

144. Answer: B

Rationale: HCAHPS (pronounced "H-caps"), also known as the CAHPS Hospital Survey, is a nationally standardized survey of patients' perspectives of their hospital experience. The survey was developed by the Centers for Medicare and Medicaid Services (CMS) in partnership with the Agency for Healthcare Research and Quality (AHRQ) and endorsed by the National Quality Forum (NQF).

145. Answer: B

Rationale: The use of excessive drugs to control behavior is considered a form of physical abuse, along with force-feeding and physical restraints.

146. Answer: B

Rationale: When an individual is covered by more than one payer source, COB ensures payment to the claimant does not exceed expenses. COB also determines which payment source pays primary. COB guidelines are voluntary.

147. Answer: D

Rationale: Adaptive families are able to adjust to crisis. They possess the ability to do the following in order to adapt:
- Be flexible
- Problem solve
- Communicate effectively
- Seek and accept help

148. Answer: A

Rationale: Concurrent Review: A method of reviewing patient care and services during a hospital stay to validate the necessity of care and to explore alternatives to inpatient care. The main purpose is to assess the need for continued hospitalization as well as the level of care provided. For example, is the ICU level of care required for this patient, or can the care be provided on a lower level unit?

149. Answer: A

Rationale: CCMC in their Glossary of Terms defines root cause analysis as a process used by healthcare providers and administrators to identify the basic or causal factors that contribute to variation in performance and outcomes or underlie the occurrence of a sentinel event (CCMC, 2017).

150. Answer: A

Rationale: Many over the counter supplements and herbs are safe to take, others can interact with medications sometimes causing severe problems. It is important for the treating physician to be aware of all treatments the client is receiving, including home remedies.

CCMC Definition and Philosophy of Case Management

Definition of Case Management

Case management is a collaborative process that assesses, plans, implements, coordinates, monitors, and evaluates the options and services required to meet the client's health and human service needs. It is characterized by advocacy, communication, and resource management and promotes quality and cost-effective interventions and outcomes.

Philosophy of Case Management

Case management is an area of specialty practice within the health and human services professions. Its underlying premise is that everyone benefits when clients(1) reach their optimum level of wellness, self-management, and functional capability.The stakeholders include the clients being served; their support systems; the health care delivery systems, including the providers of care; the employers; and the various payer sources.

Case management facilitates the achievement of client wellness and autonomy through advocacy, assessment, planning, communication, education, resource management, and service facilitation. Based on the needs and values of the client, and in collaboration with all service providers, the case manager links clients with appropriate providers and resources throughout the continuum of health and human services and care settings, while ensuring that the care provided is safe, effective, client-centered, timely, efficient, and equitable. This approach achieves optimum value and desirable outcomes for all stakeholders.

Case management services are optimized best if offered in a climate that allows direct communication among the case manager, the client, the payer, the primary care provider, and other service delivery professionals. The case manager is able to enhance these services by maintaining the client's privacy, confidentiality, health, and safety through advocacy and adherence to ethical, legal, accreditation, certification, and regulatory standards or guidelines.

Certification demonstrates that the case manager possesses the education, skills, knowledge, and experience required to render appropriate services delivered according to sound principles of practice.

(1) Client refers to the recipient of case management services. It includes, but not limited to, consumers, clients, or patients.

This material is frequently reviewed and revised as necessary. For the most current information and copy of the CCMC Code of Professional Conduct for Case Managers please visit (https://ccmcertification.org/about-ccmc/about-case-management/definition-and-philosophy-case-management).

CCMC Code of Professional Conduct

PRINCIPLES

PRINCIPLE 1: Board-Certified Case Managers (CCMs) will place the public interest above their own at all times.

PRINCIPLE 2: Board-Certified Case Managers (CCMs) will respect the rights and inherent dignity of all of their clients.

PRINCIPLE 3: Board-Certified Case Managers (CCMs) will always maintain objectivity in their relationships with clients.

PRINCIPLE 4: Board-Certified Case Managers (CCMs) will act with integrity and fidelity with clients and others.

PRINCIPLE 5: Board-Certified Case Managers (CCMs) will maintain their competency at a level that ensures their clients will receive the highest quality of service.

PRINCIPLE 6: Board-Certified Case Managers (CCMs) will honor the integrity of the CCM designation and adhere to the requirements for its use.

PRINCIPLE 7: Board-Certified Case Managers (CCMs) will obey all laws and regulations.

PRINCIPLE 8: Board-Certified Case Managers (CCMs) will help maintain the integrity of the Code, by responding to requests for public comments to review and revise the code, thus helping ensure its consistency with current practice

CCMC RULES OF CONDUCT

Violation of any of these rules may result in disciplinary action by the Commission up to and including revocation of the individual's certification.

RULE 1: A Board-Certified Case Manager (CCM) will not intentionally falsify an application or other documents.

RULE 2: A Board-Certified Case Manager (CCM) will not be convicted of a felony.

RULE 3: A Board-Certified Case Manager (CCM) will not violate the code of ethics governing the profession upon which the individual's eligibility for the CCM designation is based.

RULE 4: A Board-Certified Case Manager (CCM) will not lose the primary professional credential upon which eligibility for the CCM designation is based.

RULE 5: A Board-Certified Case Manager (CCM) will not violate or breach the Standards for Professional Conduct

RULE 6: A Board-Certified Case Manager (CCM) will not violate the rules and regulations governing the taking of the certification examination and maintenance of CCM Certification.

SCOPE OF PRACTICE FOR CASE MANAGERS

Case management is a professional, collaborative and inter-disciplinary practice. Board certification indicates that the professional case manager possesses the education, skills, moral character, and experience required to render appropriate services based on sound principles of practice.

Board-Certified Case Managers (CCMs) will practice only within the boundaries of their role or competence, based on their education, skills, and appropriate professional experience. They will not misrepresent their role or competence to clients. They will not represent the possession of the CCM credential to imply a depth of knowledge, skills, and professional capabilities greater than those demonstrated by achievement of certification.

I. UNDERLYING VALUES

- Board-Certified Case Managers (CCMs) believe that case management is a means for improving client health, wellness and autonomy through advocacy, communication, education, identification of service resources, and service facilitation.

- Board-Certified Case Managers (CCMs) recognize the dignity, worth and rights of all people.

- Board-Certified Case Managers (CCMs) understand and commit to quality outcomes for clients, appropriate use of resources, and the empowerment of clients in a manner that is supportive and objective.

- Board-Certified Case Managers (CCMs) embrace the underlying premise that when the individual(s) reaches the optimum level of wellness and functional capability, everyone benefits: the individual(s) served, their support systems, the health care delivery systems and the various reimbursement systems.
- Board-Certified Case Managers (CCMs) understand that case management is guided by the ethical principles of autonomy, beneficence, nonmaleficence, justice, and fidelity.

II. DEFINITION OF CASE MANAGEMENT

The practice of case management is a professional and collaborative process that assesses, plans, implements, coordinates, monitors, and evaluates the options and services required to meet an individual's health needs. It uses communication and available resources to promote health, quality, and cost-effective outcomes in support of the "Triple Aim," of improving the experience of care, improving the health of populations, and reducing per capita costs of health care.

III. ETHICAL ISSUES

Because case management exists in an environment that may look to it to solve or resolve various problems in the health care delivery and payor systems, case managers may often confront ethical dilemmas. Case managers must abide by the Code as well as by the professional code of ethics for their specific professional discipline for guidance and support in the resolution of these conflicts.

STANDARDS FOR BOARD-CERTIFIED CASE MANAGER (CCM) CONDUCT

SECTION 1: THE CLIENT ADVOCATE

Board-Certified Case Managers (CCMs) will serve as advocates for their clients and perform a comprehensive assessment to identify the client's needs; they will identify options and provide choices, when available and appropriate.

SECTION 2: PROFESSIONAL RESPONSIBILITY

S 1 — REPRESENTATION OF PRACTICE

Board-Certified Case Managers (CCMs) will practice only within the boundaries of their role or competence, based on their education, skills, and professional experience. They will not misrepresent their role or competence to clients.

S 2 — COMPETENCE

Case Management competence is the professional responsibility of the Board-Certified Case Manager, and is defined by educational preparation, ongoing professional development, and related work experience.

S 3 — REPRESENTATION OF QUALIFICATIONS

Board-Certified Case Managers (CCMs) will represent the possession of the CCM credential to imply the depth of knowledge, skills, and professional capabilities as intended and demonstrated by the achievement of board certification.

S 4 — LEGAL AND BENEFIT SYSTEM REQUIREMENTS

Board-Certified Case Managers (CCMs) will obey state and federal laws and the unique requirements of the various reimbursement systems by which clients are covered.

S 5 — USE OF CCM DESIGNATION

The designation of Certified Case Manager and the initials "CCM" may only be used by individuals currently certified by the Commission for Case Manager Certification. The credential is only to be used by the individual to whom it is granted, and cannot be transferred to another individual or applied to an organization.

S 6 — CONFLICT OF INTEREST

Board-Certified Case Managers (CCMs) will fully disclose any conflict of interest to all affected parties, and will not take unfair advantage of any professional relationship or exploit others for personal gain. If, after full disclosure, an objection is made by any affected party, the BoardCertified Case Manager (CCM) will withdraw from further participation in the case.

S 7 — REPORTING MISCONDUCT

Anyone possessing knowledge not protected as confidential that a Board-Certified Case Manager (CCM) may have committed a violation as to the provisions of this Code is required to promptly report such knowledge to CCMC.

S 8 — COMPLIANCE WITH PROCEEDINGS

Board-Certified Case Managers (CCMs) will assist in the process of enforcing the Code by cooperating with inquiries, participating in proceedings, and complying with the directives of the Ethics & Professional Conduct Committee.

SECTION 3: CASE MANAGER/CLIENT RELATIONSHIPS

S 9 — DESCRIPTION OF SERVICES

Board-Certified Case Managers (CCMs) will provide the necessary information to educate and empower clients to make informed decisions. At a minimum, Board-Certified Case Managers (CCMs) will provide information to clients about case management services, including a description of services, benefits, risks, alternatives and the right to refuse services. Where applicable, Board-Certified Case Managers (CCMs) will also provide the client with information about the cost of case management services prior to initiation of such services.

S 10 — RELATIONSHIPS WITH CLIENTS

Board-Certified Case Managers (CCMs) will maintain objectivity in their professional relationships, will not impose their values on their clients, and will not enter into a relationship with a client (business, personal, or otherwise) that interferes with that objectivity.

S 11 — TERMINATION OF SERVICES

Prior to the discontinuation of case management services, Board-Certified Case Managers (CCMs) will document notification of discontinuation to all relevant parties consistent with applicable statutes and regulations.

SECTION 4: CONFIDENTIALITY, PRIVACY, SECURITY AND RECORDKEEPING

S 12 — LEGAL COMPLIANCE

Board-Certified Case Managers (CCMs) will be knowledgeable about and act in accordance with federal, state, and local laws and procedures related to the scope of their practice regarding client consent, confidentiality, and the release of information.

S 13 — DISCLOSURE

Board-Certified Case Managers (CCMs) will inform the client that information obtained through the relationship may be disclosed to third parties, as prescribed by law.

S 14 — CLIENT PROTECTED HEALTH INFORMATION

As required by law, Board-Certified Case Managers (CCMs) will hold as confidential the client's protected health information, including data used for training, research, publication, and/or marketing unless a lawful, written release regarding this use is obtained from the client/legal representative.

S 15 — RECORDS

Board-Certified Case Managers (CCMs) will maintain client records, whether written, taped, computerized, or stored in any other medium, in a manner designed to ensure confidentiality.

S 16 — ELECTRONIC MEDIA

Board-Certified Case Managers (CCMs) will be knowledgeable about, and comply with, the legal requirements for privacy, confidentiality and security of the transmission and use of electronic health information. Board-Certified Case Managers (CCMs) will be accurate, honest, and unbiased in reporting the results of their professional activities to appropriate third parties.

S 17 — RECORDS: MAINTENANCE/STORAGE AND DISPOSAL

Board-Certified Case Managers (CCMs) will maintain the security of records necessary for rendering professional services to their clients and as required by applicable laws, regulations, or agency/institution procedures, (including but not limited to secured or locked files, data encryption, etc.). Subsequent to file closure, records will be maintained for the number of years consistent with jurisdictional requirements or for a longer period during which maintenance of such records is necessary or helpful to provide reasonably anticipated future services to the client. After that time, records will be destroyed in a manner assuring preservation of confidentiality, such as by shredding or other appropriate means of destruction.

SECTION 5: PROFESSIONAL RELATIONSHIPS

S 18 — TESTIMONY

Board-Certified Case Managers (CCMs), when providing testimony in a judicial or non-judicial forum, will be impartial and limit testimony to their specific fields of expertise.

S 19 — DUAL RELATIONSHIPS

Dual relationships can exist between the Board-Certified Case Manager and the client, payor, employer, friend, relative, research study and/or other entities. All dual relationships and the nature of those relationships must be disclosed by describing the role and responsibilities of the Board-Certified Case Manager (CCM).

S 20 — UNPROFESSIONAL BEHAVIOR

It is unprofessional behavior if the Board-Certified Case Manager (CCM):

- commits a criminal act;

- engages in conduct involving dishonesty, fraud, deceit, or misrepresentation;

- engages in conduct involving discrimination against a client because of race, ethnicity, religion, age, gender, sexual orientation, national origin, marital status, or disability/handicap;

- fails to maintain appropriate professional boundaries with the client;

- engages in sexually intimate behavior with a client; or accepts as a client an individual with whom the Board Certified Case Manager (CCM) has been sexually intimate;

- inappropriately discloses information about a client via social media or other means.

S 21 — FEES

Board-Certified Case Managers (CCMs) will advise the referral source/payor of their fee structure in advance of the rendering of any services and will also furnish, upon request, detailed, accurate time and expense records. No fee arrangements will be made that could compromise health care for the client.

S 22 — ADVERTISING

Board-Certified Case Managers (CCMs) who describe/ advertise services will do so in a manner that accurately informs the public of the skills and expertise being offered. Descriptions/advertisements by a Board-Certified Case Manager (CCM) will not contain false, inaccurate, misleading, out-of-context, or otherwise deceptive material or statements. If statements from former clients are used, the Board-Certified Case Manager (CCM) will have a written, signed, and dated release from these former clients. All advertising will be factually accurate and will not contain exaggerated claims as to costs and/or results.

S 23 — SOLICITATION

Board-Certified Case Managers (CCMs) will not reward, pay, or compensate any individual, company, or entity for directing or referring clients, other than as permitted by law and/or corporate policy.

S 24 — RESEARCH: LEGAL COMPLIANCE

Board-Certified Case Managers (CCMs) will plan, design, conduct, and report research in a manner that reflects cultural sensitivity; is culturally appropriate; and is consistent with pertinent ethical principles, federal and state laws, host institution regulations, and scientific standards governing research with human participants.

S 25 — RESEARCH: SUBJECT PRIVACY

Board-Certified Case Managers (CCMs) who collect data, aid in research, report research results, or make original data available will protect the identity of the respective subjects unless appropriate authorizations from the subjects have been obtained as required by law.

Footnotes:

1. Beauchamp, T. L., & Childress, J. F. (2009). Principles of Biomedical Ethics (6th ed., pp. 38-39). New York, NY: Oxford University Press.

2. Beauchamp, T. L., & Childress, J. F. (2009). Principles of Biomedical Ethics (6th ed., pp. 38-39). New York, NY: Oxford University Press.

3. Beauchamp, T. L., & Childress, J. F. (2009). Principles of Biomedical Ethics (6th ed., pp. 152-153). New York, NY: Oxford University Press.

This material is frequently reviewed and revised as necessary. For the most current information and copy of the CCMC Code of Professional Conduct for Case Managers please visit (https://ccmcertification.org/about-ccmc/code-professional-conduct).

CMSA Standards of Practice for Case Management

The following is an excerpt from the CMSA Standards of Practice for Case Management. The full standards are available on their website at: www.cmsa.org

III. Definition of Case Management

The basic concept of case management involves the timely coordination of quality services to address a client's specific needs in a cost-effective and safe manner in order to promote optimal outcomes. This can occur in a single health care setting or during the client's transitions of care throughout the care continuum. The professional case manager serves as an important facilitator among the client, family or family caregiver, the interprofessional health care team, the payer, and the community.

As demonstrated in the section on the Evolution of the Standards of Case Management, the definition of case management has evolved over a period of time; it reflects the vibrant and dynamic progression of the standards of practice.

Following more than a year of study and discussion with members of the national Case Management Task Force, the CMSA's Board of Directors approved a definition of case management in 1993.

Since that time, the CMSA Board of directors has repeatedly reviewed and analyzed the definition of case management to ensure its continued application in the dynamic health environment. The definition was modified in 2002 to reflect the process of case management outlined within the Standards. It was again revisited in 2009 and modified to further align with the practice of case management at the time. The definition was as follows (CMSA, 2009):

Case management is a collaborative process of assessment, planning, facilitation, care coordination, evaluation, and advocacy for options and services to meet an individual's and family's comprehensive health needs through communication and available resources to promote quality cost-effective outcomes.

While one may believe that the 2009 definition of case management remains appropriate today, with the recent focus on client safety, the CMSA Board of Directors has decided to explicitly reference safety in the 2016 definition:

Case Management is a collaborative process of assessment, planning, facilitation, care coordination, evaluation and advocacy for options and services to meet an individual's and family's comprehensive health needs through communication and available resources to promote patient safety, quality of care, and cost effective outcomes.

**Reprinted with permission, the Case Management Society of America, 6301 Ranch Drive, Little Rock, AR 72223, www.cmsa.org.

IV. Philosophy and Guiding Principles

A. Statement of Philosophy

A philosophy is a statement of belief and values that sets forth principles to guide a program, its meaning, its context, and the role of the individual(s) that exist in it. The CMSA's philosophy of case management articulates that:

- The underlying premise of case management is based in the fact that, when an individual reaches the optimum level of wellness and functional capability, everyone benefits: the individual client being served, the client's family or family caregiver, the health care delivery system, the reimbursement source or payer, and other involved parties such as the employer and consumer advocates.

- Professional case management serves as a means for achieving client wellness and autonomy through advocacy, ongoing communication, health education, identification of service resources, and service facilitation.

- Professional case management services are best offered in a climate that allows client's engagement and direct communication among the case manager, the client, the client's family or family caregiver, and appropriate service personnel, in order to optimize health outcomes for all concerned (CMSA, 2009).

The philosophy of case management underscores the recommendation that at-risk individuals, especially those with complex medical, behavioral, and/or psychosocial needs, be evaluated for case management intervention. The key philosophical components of case management address care that is holistic and client-centered, with mutual goals, allowing stewardship of resources for the client and the health care system including the diverse group of stakeholders. Through these efforts, case management focuses simultaneously on achieving optimal health and attaining wellness to the highest level possible for each client.

It is the philosophy of case management that when the provision of health care is effective and efficient, all parties benefit.

Case management, provided as part of a collaborative and interprofessional health care team, serves to identify options and resources which are acceptable to the client and client's family or family caregiver. This then, in turn, increases the potential for effective client's engagement in self-management, adherence to the case management plan of care, and the achievement of successful outcomes.

Case management interventions focus on improving care coordination and reducing the fragmentation of the services the recipients of care often experience especially when multiple health care providers and different care settings are involved. Taken collectively, case management interventions are intended to enhance client safety, well-being, and quality of life. These interventions carefully consider health care costs through the professional case manager's recommendations of cost-effective and efficient alternatives for care. Thus, effective case management directly and positively impacts the health care delivery system especially in realizing the goals of the "Triple Aim" which include improving the health outcomes of individuals and populations, enhancing the experience of health care, and reducing the cost of care.

B. Guiding Principles

Guiding principles are relevant and meaningful concepts that clarify or guide practice. Guiding principles for case management practice provide that professional case managers:

- Use a client-centric, collaborative partnership approach that is responsive to the individual client's culture, preferences, needs, and values.

- Facilitate client's self-determination and self-management through the tenets of advocacy, shared and informed decision-making, counseling, and health education, whenever possible.

- Use a comprehensive, holistic, and compassionate approach to care delivery which integrates a client's medical, behavioral, social, psychological, functional, and other needs.

- Practice cultural and linguistic sensitivity, and maintain current knowledge of diverse populations within their practice demographics.

- Implement evidence-based care guidelines in the care of clients, as available and applicable to the practice setting and/or client population served.

- Promote optimal client safety at the individual, organizational, and community level.

- Promote the integration of behavioral change science and principles throughout the case management process.

- Facilitate awareness of and connections with community supports and resources.

- Foster safe and manageable navigation through the health care system to enhance the client's timely access to services and the achievement of successful outcomes.

- Pursue professional knowledge and practice excellence and maintain competence in case management and health and human service delivery.

- Support systematic approaches to quality management and health outcomes improvement, implementation of practice innovations, and dissemination of knowledge and practice to the health care community.

- Maintain compliance with federal, state, and local rules and regulations, and organizational, accreditation, and certification standards.

- Demonstrate knowledge, skills, and competency in the application of case management standards of practice and relevant codes of ethics and professional conduct.

Case management guiding principles, interventions, and strategies target the achievement of optimal wellness, function, and autonomy for the client and client's family or family caregiver through advocacy, assessment, planning, communication, health education, resource management, care coordination, collaboration, and service facilitation.

The professional case manager applies these principles into practice based on the individualized needs and values of the client to assure, in collaboration with the interprofessional health care team, the provision of safe, appropriate, effective, client-centered, timely, efficient, and equitable care and services.

V. Case Management Practice Settings

Professional case management practice extends to all health care settings across the continuum of health and human services. This may include the payer, provider, government, employer, community, and client's home environment. The practice varies in degrees of complexity, intensity, urgency and comprehensiveness based on the following four factors (Powell and Tahan, 2008; Tahan and Treiger, 2017):

1. The context of the care setting such as wellness and prevention, acute, subacute and rehabilitative, skilled care, or end-of-life.

2. The health conditions and needs of the client population(s) served, and the needs of the client's family or family caregivers.

3. The reimbursement method applied, such as managed care, workers' compensation, Medicare, or Medicaid.

4. The health care professional discipline of the designated case manager such as but not limited to a registered nurse, social worker, physician, rehabilitation counselor, and disability manager.

The following is a representative list of case management practice settings; however, it is not an exhaustive reflection of where professional case managers exist today. Case managers practice in:

- Hospitals and integrated care delivery systems, including acute care, sub-acute care, long-term acute care (LTAC) facilities skilled nursing facilities (SNFs), and rehabilitation facilities.
- Ambulatory care clinics and community-based organizations, including student or university counseling and health care centers, medical and health homes, primary care practices, and federally qualified health centers.
- Corporations.
- Schools.
- Public health insurance and benefit programs such as Medicare, Medicaid, and state-funded programs.
- Private health insurance programs such as workers' compensation, occupational health, catastrophic and disability management, liability, casualty, automotive, accident and health, long-term care insurance, group health insurance, and managed care organizations.
- Independent and private case management companies.
- Government-sponsored programs such as correctional facilities, military health and Veterans Administration, and public health.
- Provider agencies and community-based facilities such as mental/behavioral health facilities, home health services, ambulatory, and day care facilities.
- Geriatric services, including residential, senior centers, assisted living facilities, and continuing care retirement communities.
- Long-term care services, including home, skilled, custodial, and community based programs.
- End-of-Life, hospice, palliative, and respite care programs
- Physician and medical group practices,

Patient Centered Medical Home (PCMH), Accountable Care Organizations (ACOs), and Physician Hospital Organizations (PHOs).
- Life care planning programs.
- Population health, wellness and prevention programs, and disease and chronic care management companies.

VI. Professional Case Management Roles and Responsibilities

It is necessary to differentiate between the terms "role," "function," and "activity" before describing the responsibilities of professional case managers. Defining these terms provides a clear and contextual understanding of the roles and responsibilities of case managers in the various practice settings.

A role is a general and abstract term that refers to a set of behaviors and expected consequences that are associated with one's position in a social structure. A function is a grouping or a set of specific tasks or activities within the role. An activity is a discrete action, behavior or task a person performs to address the expectations of the role assumed (Tahan and Campagna, 2010).

A role consists of several functions and each function is described through a list of specific and related activities. These descriptions constitute what is commonly known as a "job description" (Tahan and Campagna, 2010). The roles professional case managers assume may vary based on the same four factors described earlier in the section entitled, Case Management Practice Settings.

The professional case manager performs the primary functions of assessment, planning, facilitation, coordination, monitoring, evaluation, and advocacy. Integral to these functions is collaboration and ongoing communication with the client, client's family or family caregiver, and other health care professionals involved in the client's care. Nationally recognized professional associations and specialty certifying bodies have identified key responsibilities of case managers through expert opinions, practice analyses, and roles and functions research.

It is not the intent of the *Standards of Practice for Case Management* to parallel these key responsibilities. The Standards broadly define major functions involved in the case management process to achieve desired outcomes. The specific roles and responsibilities of professional case managers may vary based on their health discipline background and the environment or care setting they practice in.

Successful care outcomes cannot be achieved without the specialized skills, knowledge, and competencies professional case managers apply throughout the case management process. These include, but are not limited to, motivational interviewing and positive relationship-building; effective written and verbal communication; negotiation and brokerage of services; cost-conscious allocation of resources; knowledge of contractual health insurance or risk arrangements; client activation, empowerment, and engagement; the ability to effect change, perform ongoing evaluation and critical analysis; and the skill to plan, organize, and manage competing priorities effectively.

To facilitate effective and competent performance, the professional case manager should demonstrate knowledge of health insurance and funding sources, health care services, human behavior dynamics, health care delivery and financing systems, community resources, ethical and evidence-based practice, applicable laws and regulations, clinical standards and outcomes, and health information technology and digital media relevant to case management practice. The skills and knowledge base of a professional case manager may be applied to individual clients such as in the hospital setting, or to groups of clients such as in disease, chronic care, or population health management models. Often case managers execute their responsibilities across settings, providers, over time, and beyond the boundaries of a single episode of care. They also employ the use of health and information technology and tools.

The role functions of professional case managers may include, but are not limited to, the following:

- Considering predictive modeling, screening, and other data, where appropriate, in deciding whether a client would benefit from case management services.

- Conducting an assessment of the client's health, physical, functional, behavioral, psychological, and social needs, including health literacy status and deficits, self-management abilities and engagement in taking care of own health, availability of psychosocial support systems including family caregivers, and socioeconomic background. The assessment leads to the development and implementation of a client-specific case management plan of care in collaboration with the client and family or family caregiver, and other essential health care professionals

- Identifying target care goals in collaboration with the client, client's family or family caregiver, and other members of the health care team. Securing client's agreement on the target goals and desired outcomes.

- Planning the care interventions and needed resources with the client, family or family caregiver, the primary care provider, other health care professionals, the payer, and the community-based agents, to maximize the client's health care responses, quality, safety, cost-effective outcomes, and optimal care experience.

- Facilitating communication and coordination among members of the interprofessional health care team, and involving the client in the decision-making process in order to minimize fragmentation in the services provided and prevent the risk for unsafe care and suboptimal outcomes.

- Collaborating with other health care professionals and support service providers across care settings, levels of care, and professional disciplines, with special attention to safe transitions of care.

- Coordinating care interventions, referrals to specialty providers and community-based support services, consults, and resources across involved health providers and care settings.

- Communicating on an ongoing basis with the client, client's family or family caregiver, other involved health care professionals and support service providers, and assuring that all are well-informed and current on the case management plan of care and services.

- Educating the client, the family or family caregiver, and members of the interprofessional health care team about treatment options, community resources, health insurance benefits, psychosocial and financial concerns, and case management services, in order to make timely and informed care-related decisions.

- Counseling and empowering the client to problem-solve by exploring options of care, when available, and alternative plans, when necessary, to achieve desired outcomes.

- Completing indicated notifications for and pre-authorizations of services, medical necessity reviews, and concurrent or retrospective communications, based on payer's requirements and utilization management procedures.

- Ensuring the appropriate allocation, use, and coordination of health care services and resources while striving to improve safety and quality of care, and maintain cost effectiveness on a case-by-case basis.

- Identifying barriers to care and client's engagement in own health; addressing these barriers to prevent suboptimal care outcomes.

- Assisting the client in the safe transitioning of care to the next most appropriate level, setting, and/or provider.

- Striving to promote client self-advocacy, independence, and self-determination, and the provision of client-centered and culturally-appropriate care.

- Advocating for both the client and the payer to facilitate positive outcomes for the client, the interprofessional health care team, and the payer. However, when a conflict arises, the needs of the client must be the number one priority.

- Evaluating the value and effectiveness of case management plans of care, resource allocation, and service provision while applying outcomes measures reflective of organizational policies and expectations, accreditation standards, and regulatory requirements.

- Engaging in performance improvement

activities with the goal of improving client's access to timely care and services, and enhancing the achievement of target goals and desired outcomes.

VII. Components of the Case Management Process

The case management process is carried out within the ethical and legal realms of a case manager's scope of practice, using critical thinking and evidence-based knowledge. The overarching themes in the case management process include the activities described below.

Note that the case management process is cyclical and recurrent, rather than linear and unidirectional. For example, key functions of the professional case manager, such as communication, facilitation, coordination, collaboration, and advocacy, occur throughout all the steps of the case management process and in constant contact with the client, client's family or family caregiver, and other members of the interprofessional health care team. Primary steps in the case management process include:

1. Client Identification, Selection and Engagement in Professional Case Management:

- Focus on screening clients identified or referred by other professionals for case management to determine appropriateness for and benefits from services.

- Engagement of the client and family or family caregiver in the process.

- Obtaining consent for case management services as part of the case initiation process.

2. Assessment and Opportunity Identification:

- Assessment begins after screening, identification and engagement in case management. It involves data gathering, analysis, and synthesis of information for the purpose of developing a client-centric case management plan of care.

- Assessment helps establish the client-case manager's relationship and the client's readiness to engage in own health and well-being. It requires the use of effective communication skills such as active listening, meaningful conversation, motivational interviewing, and use of open-ended questions.

- Care needs and opportunities are identified through analysis of the assessment findings and determination of identified needs, barriers, and/or gaps in care.

- Assessment is an ongoing process occurring intermittently, as needed, to determine efficacy of the case management plan of care and client's progress toward achieving target goals.

- Assessment should cover medical, behavioral health, substance use and abuse and social determinants of health.

3. Development of the Case Management Plan of Care:

- The case management plan of care is a structured, dynamic tool used to document the opportunities, interventions, and expected goals, the professional case manager applies during the client's engagement in case management services. It includes:

  - Identified care needs, barriers and opportunities for collaboration with the client, family and/or family caregiver, and members of the interprofessional care team in order to provide more effective integrated care;

  - Prioritized goals and/or outcomes to be achieved; and

  - Interventions or actions needed to reach the goals.

- Client and/or client's family or family caregiver input and participation in the development of the case management plan of care is essential to promote client-centered care and maximize potential for achieving the target goals.

4. Implementation and Coordination of the Case Management Plan of Care:

- The case management plan of care is put into action by facilitating the coordination of care, services, resources, and health education specified in the planned interventions.

- Effective care coordination requires ongoing communication and collaboration with the client and/or client's family or family caregiver, as well as the provider and the entire interprofessional health care team.

5. Monitoring and Evaluation of the Case Management Plan of Care:

- Ongoing follow-up with the client, family and/or family caregiver and evaluation of the client's status, goals, and outcomes.

- Monitoring activities include assessing client's progress with planned interventions

- Evaluating if care goals and interventions remain appropriate, relevant, and realistic.

- Determining if any revisions or modifications are needed to the care needs, goals, or interventions specified in the client's case management plan of care

6. Closure of the Professional Case Management Services:

- Bringing mutually-agreed upon closure to the client-case manager relationship and engagement in case management.

- Case closure focuses on discontinuing the professional case management services when the client has attained the highest level of functioning and recovery, the best possible outcomes, or when the needs and desires of the client have changed.

VIII. Standards of Professional Case Management Practice

A. STANDARD: CLIENT SELECTION PROCESS FOR PROFESSIONAL CASE MANAGEMENT SERVICES

The professional case manager should screen clients referred for case management services to identify those who are appropriate for and most likely to benefit from case management services available within a particular practice setting.

How Demonstrated:

- Documentation of consistent use of the client selection process within the organization's policies and procedures.

- Use of screening criteria as appropriate to select a client for inclusion in case management. Examples of screening criteria may include, but are not limited to:

    - Barriers to accessing care and services

    - Advanced age

    - Catastrophic or life-altering conditions

    - Chronic, complex, or terminal conditions

    - Concerns regarding self-management ability and adherence to health regimens

    - Developmental disabilities

    - End-of-life or palliative care

    - History of abuse or neglect

    - History of mental illness, substance use, suicide risk, or crisis intervention

    - Financial hardships

    - Housing and transportation needs

    - Lack of adequate social support including family caregiver support

    - Low educational levels

    - Low health literacy, reading literacy, or numeracy literacy levels

    - Impaired functional status and/or cognitive deficits

    - Multiple admissions, readmissions, and emergency department (ED) visits

    - Multiple providers delivering care and/or no primary care provider

    - Polypharmacy and medication adherence needs

    - Poor nutritional status

    - Poor pain control

    - Presence of actionable gaps in care and services

    - Previous home health and durable medical equipment usage

    - Results of established predictive modeling analysis and/or health risk screening tools indicative of need for case management

    - Risk taking behaviors

- Recognition that a professional case manager may receive pre-screened client referrals from various sources, including (but not limited to) direct referrals from health care professionals and system-generated flags, alerts, or triggers. In these situations, the case manager should document the referral source and why the client is appropriate for case management services.

B. STANDARD: ASSESSMENT

The professional case manager should complete a thorough individualized client centered assessment that takes into account the unique cultural and linguistic needs of that client including client's family or family caregiver as appropriate.

It is recognized that an assessment:

- is a process, that focuses on evolving client needs identified by the case manager over the duration of the professional relationship and across the transitions of care;

- involves each client and/or the client's family or family caregiver as appropriate, and;

- is inclusive of the medical, cognitive, behavioral, social, and functional domains, as pertinent to the practice setting (Kathol, Perez, & Cohen, 2010) the client uses to access care.

How Demonstrated:

- Documented client assessments using standardized tools, both electronic and written, when appropriate. The assessment may include, but is not limited to the following components:

Medical

- Presenting health status and conditions
- Medical history including use of prescribed or over the counter medications and herbal therapies
- Relevant treatment history
- Prognosis
- Nutritional status

Cognitive and Behavioral

- Mental health
  - History of substance use
  - Depression risk screening
  - History of treatment including prescribed or over the counter medications and herbal therapies
- Cognitive functioning
  - Language and communication preferences, needs, or limitations
- Client strengths and abilities
  - Self-care and self-management capability
  - Readiness to change
- Client professional and educational focus
  - Vocational and/or educational interests
  - Recreational and leisure pursuits
- Self-Management and Engagement Status
  - Health literacy
  - Health activation level
  - Knowledge of health condition
  - Knowledge of and adherence to plan of care
  - Medication management and adherence
  - Learning and technology capabilities

Social

- Psychosocial status
  - Family or family caregiver dynamics

- Caregiver resources: availability and degree of involvement
- Environmental and residential
- Financial Circumstances
- Client beliefs, values, needs, and preferences including cultural and spiritual
- Access to care
  - Health insurance status and availability of health care benefits
  - Health care providers involved in client's care
  - Barriers to getting care and resources
- Safety concerns and needs
  - History of neglect, abuse, violence, or trauma
  - Safety of the living situation
- Advanced directives planning and availability of documentation
- Pertinent legal situations (e.g. custody, marital discord, and immigration status)

Functional

- Client priorities and self-identified care goals
- Functional status
- Transitional or discharge planning needs and services, if applicable
  - Health care services currently receiving or recently received in the home setting
  - Skilled nursing, home health aide, durable medical equipment (DME), or other relevant services
  - Transportation capability and constraints
  - Follow-up care (e.g., primary care, specialty care, and appointments)
  - Safety and appropriateness of home or residential environment
- Reassessment of the client's condition, response to the case management plan of care and interventions, and progress toward achieving care goals and target outcomes.

- Documentation of resource utilization and cost management, provider options, and available health and behavioral care benefits.
- Evidence of relevant information and data required for the client's thorough assessment and obtained from multiple sources including, but not limited to:
  - Client interviews;
  - Initial and ongoing assessments and care summaries available in the client's health record and across the transitions of care;
  - Family caregivers (as appropriate), physicians, providers, and other involved members of the interprofessional health care team;
  - Past medical records available as appropriate; and
  - Claims and administrative data.

C. STANDARD: CARE NEEDS AND OPPORTUNITIES IDENTIFICATION

The professional case manager should identify the client's care needs or opportunities that would benefit from case management interventions.

How Demonstrated:

- Documented agreement among the client and/or client's family or family caregiver, and other providers and organizations regarding the care needs and opportunities identified.
- Documented identification of opportunities for intervention, such as:
  - Lack of established, evidenced-based plan of care with specific goals
  - Over-utilization or under-utilization of services and resources
  - Use of multiple providers and/or agencies
  - Lack of integrated care
  - Use of inappropriate services or level of care
  - Lack of a primary provider or any provider

- Non-adherence to the case management plan of care (e.g. medication adherence) which may be associated with the following:
  - Low reading level
  - Low health literacy and/or numeracy
  - Low health activation levels
  - Language and communication barriers
- Lack of education or understanding of:
  - Disease process
  - Current condition(s)
  - The medication list
  - Substance use and abuse
  - Social determinants of health
- Lack of ongoing evaluation of the client's limitations in the following aspects of health condition:
  - Medical
  - Cognitive and Behavioral
  - Social
  - Functional
- Lack of support from the client's family or family caregiver especially when under stress
- Financial barriers to adherence of the case management plan of care
- Determination of patterns of care or behavior that may be associated with increased severity of condition
- Compromised client safety
- Inappropriate discharge or delay from other levels of care
- High cost injuries or illnesses
- Complications related to medical, psychosocial or functional condition or needs
- Lack of support from the client's family or family caregiver especially when under stress
- Frequent transitions between care settings or providers
- Poor or no coordination of care between settings or providers

D. STANDARD: PLANNING

The professional case manager, in collaboration with the client, client's family or family caregiver, and other members of the interprofessional health care team, where appropriate, should identify relevant care goals and interventions to manage the client's identified care needs and opportunities. The case manager should also document these in an individualized case management plan of care.

How Demonstrated:

- Documented relevant, comprehensive information and data using analysis of assessment findings, client and/or client's family or family caregiver interviews, input from the client's interprofessional healthcare team, and other methods as needed to develop an individualized case management plan of care.

- Documented client and/or client's family or family caregiver participation in the development of the written case management plan of care.

- Documented client agreement with the case management plan of care, including agreement with target goals, expected outcomes, and any changes or additions to the plan.

- Recognized client's needs, preferences, and desired role in decision-making concerning the development of the case management plan of care.

- Validated that the case management plan of care is consistent with evidence-based practice, when such guidelines are available and applicable, and that it continues to meet the client's changing needs and health condition.

- Established measurable goals and outcome indicators expected to be achieved within specified time frames. These measures could include clinical as well as non-clinical domains of outcomes management. For example, access to care, cost-effectiveness of care, safety and quality of care, and client's experience of care.

- Evidence of supplying the client, client's family, or family caregiver with information and resources necessary to make informed decisions.

- Promoted awareness of client care goals, outcomes, resources, and services included in the case management plan of care.

- Adherence to payer expectations with respect to how often to contact and reevaluate the client, redefine long and short term goals, or update the case management plan of care.

E. STANDARD: MONITORING

The professional case manager should employ ongoing assessment with appropriate documentation to measure the client's response to the case management plan of care.

How Demonstrated:

- Documented ongoing collaboration with the client, family or family caregiver, providers, and other pertinent stakeholders, so that the client's response to interventions is reviewed and incorporated into the case management plan of care.

- Awareness of circumstances necessitatin revisions to the case management plan of care, such as changes in the client's condition, lack of response to the case management interventions, change in the client's preferences, transitions across care settings and/o providers, and barriers to care and services.

- Evidence that the plan of care continues to be reviewed and is appropriate, understood, accepted by client and/or client's family or family caregiver, and documented.

- Ongoing collaboration with the client, family or family caregiver, providers, and other pertinent stakeholders regarding any revisions to the plan of care.

F. STANDARD: OUTCOMES

The professional case manager, through a thorough individualized client centered assessment, should maximize the client's health, wellness, safety, physical functioning, adaptation, health knowledge, coping with chronic illness, engagement, and self-management abilities.

How Demonstrated:

- Created a case management plan of care based on the thorough individualized client-centered assessment.

- Achieved through quality and cost-efficient case management services, client's satisfaction with the experience of care, shared and informed decision-making, and engagement in own health and health care.

- Evaluated the extent to which the goals and target outcomes documented in the case management plan of care have been achieved.

- Demonstrated efficacy, efficiency, quality, safety, and cost-effectiveness of the professional case manager's interventions in achieving the goals documented in the case management plan of care and agreed upon with the client and/or client's family caregiver.

- Measured and reported impact of the case management plan of care.

- Applied evidence-based adherence guidelines, standardized tools and proven care processes. These can be used to measure the client's preference for, and understanding of:

  - The proposed case management plan of care and needed resources;

  - Motivation to change and demonstrate healthy lifestyle behavior; and

  - Importance of availability of engaged client, family or family caregiver.

- Applied evidence-based guidelines relevant to the care of specific client populations.

- Evaluated client and/or client's family or family caregiver experience with case management services.

- Used national performance measures for transitional care and care coordination such as those endorsed by the regulatory, accreditation, and certification agencies, and health-related professional associations to ultimately enhance quality, efficiency and optimal client experience

G. STANDARD: CLOSURE OF PROFESSIONAL CASE MANAGEMENT SERVICES

The professional case manager should appropriately complete closure of professional case management services based upon established case closure guidelines. The extent of applying these guidelines may differ in various case management practice and/or care settings.

How Demonstrated:

- Achieved care goals and target outcomes, including those self-identified by the client and/or client's family or family caregiver.

- Identified reasons for and appropriateness of closure of case management services, such as:

  - Reaching maximum benefit from case management services;

  - Change of health care setting which warrants the transition of the client's care to another health care provider(s) and/or setting;

  - The employer or purchaser of case management services requests the closure of case management;

  - Services no longer meet program or benefit eligibility requirements;

  - Client refuses further case management services;

  - Determination by the professional case manager that he/she is no longer able to provide appropriate case management services because of situations such as a client's ongoing disengagement in self-management and unresolved non-adherence to the case management plan of care;

  - Death of the client;

  - There is a conflict of interest; and

- When a dual relationship raises ethical concerns.
- Evidence of agreement for closure of case management services by the client, family or family caregiver, payer, professional case manager, and/or other appropriate parties.
- Evidence that when a barrier to closure of professional case management services arises, the case manager has discussed the situation with the appropriate stakeholders and has reached agreement on a plan to resolve the barrier.
- Documented reasonable notice for closure of professional case management services and actual closure that is based upon the facts and circumstances of each individual client's case and care outcomes supporting case closure. Evidence should show verbal and/or written notice of case closure to the client and other directly involved healthcare professionals and support service providers.
- Evidence of client education about service and/or funding resources provided by the professional case manager to addressany further needs of the client upon case closure.
- Completed transition of care handover to health care providers at the next level of care, where appropriate, with permission from client, and inclusive of communication of relevant client information and continuity of the case management plan of care to optimize client care outcomes.

H. STANDARD: FACILITATION, COORDINATION, AND COLLABORATION

The professional case manager should facilitate coordination, communication, and collaboration with the client, client's family or family caregiver, involved members of the interprofessional healthcare team, and other stakeholders, in order to achieve target goals and maximize positive client care outcomes.

How Demonstrated:

- Recognition of the professional case manager's role and practice setting in relation to those of other providers and organizations involved in the provision of care and case management services to the client.
- Developing and sustaining proactive client-centered relationships through open communication with the client, client's family or family caregiver, and other relevant stakeholders, to maximize outcomes and enhance client's safety and optimal care experience.
- Evidence of facilitation, coordination, and collaboration to support the transitions of care, including:
  - Transfers of clients to the most appropriate health care provider or care setting are coordinated in a timely and complete manner.
  - Documentation reflective of the collaborative and transparent communication between the professional case manager and other health care team members, especially during each transition to another level of care within or outside of the client's current setting.
  - Use of the case management plan of care, target goals, and client's needs and preferences to guide the facilitation and coordination of services and collaboration among members of the interprofessional health care team, client and client's family or family caregiver.
- Adherence to client privacy and confidentiality mandates during all aspects of facilitation, coordination, communication, and collaboration within and outside the client's care setting.
- Use of special techniques and strategies such as motivational interviewing, mediation, and negotiation, to facilitate transparent communication and building of effective relationships.
- Coordination and implementation of the use of problem-solving skills and techniques to reconcile potentially differing points of view.
- Evidence of collaboration that optimizes client outcomes; this may include working with community, local and state resources,

primary care providers, members of the interprofessional health care team, the payer, and other relevant stakeholders.

- Evidence of collaborative efforts to maximize adherence to regulatory and accreditation standards within the professional case manager's practice and employment setting.

I. STANDARD: QUALIFICATIONS FOR PROFESSIONAL CASE MANAGERS

The professional case manager should maintain competence in her/his area(s) of practice by having one of the following:

- Current, active and unrestricted licensure or certification in a health or human services discipline that allows the professional to conduct an assessment independently as permitted within the scope of practice of the discipline; or

- In the case of an individual who practices in a state that does not require licensure or certification, the individual must have a baccalaureate or graduate degree in social work or another health or human services field that promotes the physical, psychosocial, and/or vocational well-being of the persons being served. The degree must be from an institution that is fully accredited by a nationally recognized educational accreditation organization, and;

- The individual must have completed a supervised field experience in case management, health or behavioral health as part of the degree requirements.

How Demonstrated:

- Possession of the education, experience, and expertise required for the professional case manager's area(s) of practice.

- Compliance with national, state, and/or local laws and regulations that apply to the jurisdiction(s) and discipline(s) in which the professional case manager practices.

- Maintenance of competence through participation in relevant and ongoing continuing education, certification, academic study, and internship programs.

- Practicing within the professional case manager's area(s) of expertise, making timely and appropriate referrals to, and seeking consultation with, others when needed.

Supervision

The professional case manager acts in a supervisory and/or leadership role of other personnel who are unable to function independently due to limitations of license and/or education.

Due to the variation in academic degrees and other educational requirements, it is recommended that individuals interested in pursuing a professional case management career seek guidance as to the appropriate educational preparation and academic degree necessary to practice case management. These interested individuals may seek the Case Management Society of America, American Nurses Association, or Commission for Case Manager Certification, or other relevant professional organizations for further advice and guidance.

NOTE: *Social workers who are prepared at the CMSA Standards of Practice for Case Management 27 Master's in Social Work (MSW) degree level and educated under a program that would preclude them from sitting for licensure (where required) or practice at the clinical level should consult with their state licensing board to determine if additional education and/or practicum hours are required.*

J. STANDARD: LEGAL

The professional case manager shall adhere to all applicable federal, state, and local laws and regulations, which have full force and effect of law, governing all aspects of case management practice including, but not limited to, client privacy and confidentiality rights. It is the responsibility of the professional case manager to work within the scope of his/her license and/or underlying profession.

NOTE: *In the event that the professional case manager's employer policies or those of other entities are in conflict with applicable legal requirements, the case manager should understand that the law prevails. In these situations, case managers should seek clarification of questions or concerns from an appropriate and reliable expert resource, such as a legal counsel, compliance officer, or an appropriate government agency.*

1. Standard: Confidentiality and Client Privacy

The professional case manager should adhere to federal, state, and local laws, as well as policies and procedures, governing client privacy and confidentiality, and should act in a manner consistent with the client's best interest in all aspects of communication and recordkeeping whether through traditional paper records and/or electronic health records (EHR).

NOTE: *Federal law preempts (supersedes) state and local law and provides a minimum mandatory national standard; states may enlarge client rights, but not reduce them. For those who work exclusively on federal enclaves or on tribal lands, any issues of concern should direct them to the licensing authority and/or federal law.*

How Demonstrated:

- Demonstration of up-to-date knowledge of, and adherence to, applicable laws and regulations concerning confidentiality, privacy, and protection of the client's medical information.
- Evidence of a good faith effort to obtain the client's written acknowledgement that she/he has received notice of privacy rights and practices.

2. Standard: Consent for Professional Case Management Services

The professional case manager should obtain appropriate and informed consent before the implementation of case management services.

How Demonstrated:

- Evidence that the client and/or client's family or family caregiver have been thoroughly informed with regard to:
  - Proposed case management process and services relating to the client's health condition(s) and needs;
  - Possible benefits and costs of such services;
  - Alternatives to proposed services;
  - Potential risks and consequences of proposed services and alternatives; and
  - Client's right to decline the proposed case management services and awareness of potential risks and consequences of such decision.
- Evidence that the information was communicated in a client-sensitive manner, which is intended to permit the client to make voluntary and informed choices.
- Documented informed consent where client consent is a prerequisite to the provision of case management services.

K. ETHICS

The professional case manager should behave and practice ethically, and adhere to the tenets of the code of ethics that underlie her/his professional credentials (e.g., nursing, social work, and rehabilitation counseling).

How Demonstrated:

- Awareness of the five basic ethical principles and how they are applied. These are:
  - Beneficence (to do good),
  - Nonmaleficence (to do no harm),
  - Autonomy (to respect individuals' rights to make their own decisions),
  - Justice (to treat others fairly), and
  - Fidelity (to follow-through and to keep promises).
- Recognition that:
  - A primary obligation is to the clients cared for, with
  - A secondary obligation is engagement in and maintenance of respectful relationships with coworkers, employers, and other professionals.
  - Laws, rules, policies, insurance benefits, and regulations are sometimes in conflict with ethical

principles. In such situations, the professional case manager is bound to address the conflicts to the best of her/his abilities and/or seek appropriate consultation.

- All clients are unique individuals and the professional case manager engages them without regard to gender identity, race or ethnicity, and practice, religious, other cultural preferences, or socioeconomic status.

● Maintained policies that are universally respectful of the integrity and worth of each person.

L. STANDARD: ADVOCACY

The professional case manager should advocate for the client, client's family or family caregiver, at the service delivery, benefits administration, and policy-making levels. The case manager is uniquely positioned as an expert in care coordination and advocacy for health policy change to improve access to quality, safe, and cost-effective services.

How Demonstrated:

● Documentation demonstrating:

- Promotion of the client's self-determination, informed and shared decision-making, autonomy, growth, and self-advocacy.

- Education of other health care and service providers in recognizing and respecting the needs, strengths, and goals of the client.

- Facilitation of client access to necessary and appropriate services while educating the client and family or family caregiver about resource availability within practice settings.

- Recognition, prevention, and elimination of disparities in accessing high-quality care and experiencing optimal client health care outcomes, as related to race, ethnicity, national origin, and migration background; sex and marital status; age, religion, and political belief; physical, mental, or cognitive disability; gender identity or gender expression; or other cultural factors.

- Advocacy for expansion or establishment of services and for client-centered changes in organizational and governmental policy.

● Ensuring a culture of safety by engagement in quality improvement initiatives in the workplace.

● Encouraging the establishment of client, family and/or family caregiver advisory councils to improve client-centered care standards within the organization.

● Joining relevant professional organizations in call to action campaigns, whenever possible, to improve the quality of care and reduce health disparities.

● Recognition that client advocacy can sometimes conflict with a need to balance cost constraints and limited resources Documentation indicates that the professional case manager has weighed decisions with the intent to uphold client advocacy, whenever possible.

M. STANDARD: CULTURAL COMPETENCY

The professional case manager should maintain awareness of and be responsive to cultural and linguistic diversity of the demographics of her/his work setting and to the specific client and/or caregiver needs.

How Demonstrated:

● Evidence of communicating in an effective, respectful, and sensitive manner, and in accordance with the client's cultural and linguistic context.

● Assessments, goal-setting, and development of a case management plan of care to accommodate each client's cultural and linguistic needs and preference of services.

● Identified appropriate resources to enhance the client's access to care and improve healthcare outcomes. These may include the use of interpreters and health educational materials which apply language and format demonstrative of understanding of the client's cultural and linguistic communication patterns, including but not limited to speech volume, context, tone, kinetics, space, and other similar verbal/non-verbal communication patterns.

- Pursuit of professional education to maintain and advance one's level of cultural competence and effectiveness while working with diverse client populations.

N. STANDARD: RESOURCE MANAGEMENT AND STEWARDSHIP

The professional case manager should integrate factors related to quality, safety, access, and cost-effectiveness in assessing, planning, implementing, monitoring, and evaluating health resources for client care.

How Demonstrated:

- Documented evaluation of safety, effectiveness, cost, and target outcomes when designing a case management plan of care to promote the ongoing care needs of the client.

- Evidence of follow-through on the objectives of the case management plan of care which are based on the ongoing care needs of the client and the competency, knowledge, and skills of the professional case manager.

- Application of evidence-based guidelines and practices, when appropriate, in recommending resource allocation and utilization options.

- Evidence of linking the client and family or family caregiver with cultural and linguistically appropriate resources to meet the needs and goals identified in the case management plan of care.

- Documented communication with the client and family or family caregiver about the length of time for availability of a necessary resource, potential and actual financial responsibility associated with a resource, and the range of outcomes associated with resource utilization.

- Documented communication with the client and other interprofessional healthcare team members, especially during care transitions or when there is a significant change in the client's situation.

- Evidence of promoting the most effective and efficient use of health care services and financial resources.

- Documentation which reflects that the intensity of case management services rendered corresponds with the needs of the client.

O. STANDARD: PROFESSIONAL RESPONSIBILITIES AND SCHOLARSHIP

The professional case manager should engage in scholarly activities and maintain familiarity with current knowledge, competencies, case management-related research, and evidencesupported care innovations. The professional case manager should also identify best practices in case management and health care service delivery, and apply such in transforming practice, as appropriate.

How Demonstrated:

- Incorporation of current and relevant research findings into one's practice, including policies, procedures, care protocols or guidelines, and workflow processes, and as applicable to the care setting.

- Efficient retrieval and appraisal of research evidence that is pertinent to one's practice and client population served.

- Proficiency in the application of researchrelated and evidence-based practice tools and terminologies.

- Ability to distinguish peer-reviewed materials (e.g., research results, publications) and apply preference to such work in practice, as available and appropriate.

- Accountability and responsibility for own professional development and advancement.

- Participation in ongoing training and/ or educational opportunities (e.g., conferences, webinars, academic

academic programs) to maintain and expand one's skills, knowledge and competencies.

- Participation in research activities which support quantification and definition of valid and reliable outcomes, especially those that demonstrate the value of case management services and their impact on the individual client and population health.

- Identification and evaluation of best practices and innovative case management interventions.

- Leveraging opportunities in the employment setting to conduct innovativeperformance improvement projects and formally report on their results.

- Dissemination, through publication and/ or presentation at conferences, of practice innovations, research findings, evidencebased practices, and quality or performance improvement efforts.

- Membership in professional case management-related associations and involvement in local, regional, or national committees and taskforces.

- Mentoring and coaching of less experienced case managers, other interprofessional health care team members, and providers.

*Reprinted with permission, the Case Management Society of America, 6301 Ranch Drive, Little Rock, AR 72223, www.cmsa.org.

Index

coordinates 14, 16, 20, 103, 132, 349, 362, 364

coordination 3, 15, 16, 20, 23, 48, 50, 102, 105, 106, 120, 189, 199, 200, 205, 206, 213, 223, 225, 290, 293, 338, 367, 368, 369, 370, 371, 372, 373, 376, 378, 379, 382

Coordination of Benefits (COB) 64

Coordination of care 24

CoP 190, 279

copayment 77, 78, 79, 81, 83, 93, 109, 127

coping skills 164, 170, 311, 343

Core Components of Case Management 3

Core Measures 207, 336, 359

Cost-benefit 215, 217, 314, 325

cost-benefit analysis 21, 234, 344

cost-effective 14, 16, 59, 95, 105, 115, 147, 189, 317, 346, 347, 349, 362, 364, 367, 368, 371, 382

cost savings 217, 218, 219, 306, 307, 309, 340

cost-sharing 81, 83, 132, 287, 288

counseling 51, 52, 53, 63, 81, 88, 93, 119, 138, 159, 160, 161, 164, 170, 236, 241, 242, 270, 288, 325, 351, 355, 369, 370, 381

counselors 40, 241

CQMs 204

credentialing 199, 200

critical access hospitals 76

cultural assessment 169

cultural beliefs 14, 169, 185, 335, 358

cultural competence 168, 268, 383

cultural competency 169

Current Procedural Terminology (CPT) 100, 101

custodial care 79, 117, 131, 348

Custodial care 118, 348

D

deductible 77, 78, 79, 81, 82, 83, 85, 109, 126, 308,

318, 341, 347

Defense Health Agency (DHA) 91

delivery system 91, 107, 108, 109, 291, 304, 368

Delivery System 107, 108

Department of Veterans Affairs (VA) 92, 93

dependent 54, 61, 65, 72, 73, 74, 249, 319

depression 32, 37, 52, 55, 63, 123, 129, 148, 151, 159, 170, 172, 180, 201, 206, 255, 287, 311, 319, 335, 343

developmental 32, 33, 35, 236, 240, 242

Developmental Task 34, 35, 36, 37, 38, 39

diagnosis-related group (DRG) 96

Diagnostic and Statistical Manual of Mental Disorders 101, 149, 164, 308, 314, 341, 345

Diagnostic and Statistical Manual of Mental Disorders (DSM) 101

Diagnostic and Statistical Manual of Mental Disorders (DSM-5) 149, 308, 341

dietitian 55

disability 24, 41, 47, 63, 64, 67, 68, 69, 70, 73, 75, 76, 78, 89, 90, 93, 126, 156, 157, 199, 222, 236, 242, 243, 244, 246, 248, 250, 255, 280, 281, 282, 283, 292, 307, 311, 320, 329, 335, 340, 342, 349, 356, 366, 369, 370, 382

Disability Case Management 40

disabled 41, 54, 60, 66, 67, 73, 89, 90, 127, 158, 163, 242, 285, 348

disabled employee 41

disabled workers 67, 89, 348

discharge 17, 20, 21, 22, 28, 40, 46, 48, 93, 96, 101, 129, 145, 187, 208, 212, 239, 255, 273, 286, 290, 293, 338, 375, 376

Discharge planning 24, 25, 273

Discharge Planning 21, 331

disease-based agencies 40

Disease management 24

document 48, 52, 77, 118, 172, 216, 217, 218, 233, 238, 248, 257, 265, 269, 273, 277, 293, 300,

plan of care 18, 19, 21, 31, 33, 52, 53, 99, 137, 143, 145, 157, 180, 218, 268, 329, 334, 337, 340, 346, 354, 368, 371, 372, 373, 375, 376, 377, 378, 379, 382, 383

Point of Service Plans (POSs) 108

Point-of-Service (POS) 111

population 18, 32, 33, 42, 99, 100, 103, 106, 108, 145, 168, 200, 206, 220, 223, 316, 369, 371, 383, 384

population health 42, 99, 100, 200, 206, 223, 371, 384

Population health 99, 213, 370

population management 18

post-transition services 20

PPS 54, 75, 95, 96, 98, 338

practice guidelines 209, 224

Practice Standards 3, 7, 263, 298

preauthorization 114

precertification 25, 115

precertifications 114

Predictive modeling 222, 223, 327, 353

Preferred Provider Organizations (PPOs) 108, 110

prescription 44, 45, 72, 77, 81, 84, 88, 109, 131, 160, 164, 282, 293, 315, 317, 328, 347, 354

prevention 16, 23, 33, 35, 99, 105, 138, 162, 180, 206, 213, 221, 350, 369, 370, 382

preventive care 38, 62, 64, 91, 110, 112, 141, 171, 308

primary care 15, 16, 46, 47, 48, 103, 106, 107, 112, 153, 206, 291, 292, 335, 362, 370, 371, 374, 375, 380

Primary Care Provider 110

prior-authorization 72

professional standards 272, 277, 331

Prospective Payment 75, 94, 95, 96, 97, 98, 215, 290

Prospective Payment System (PPS) 75, 95, 98

Prospective reviews 114

prosthetic 240, 251, 259

protected health information (PHI) 283

provider 14, 20, 23, 40, 42, 47, 48, 50, 71, 80, 81, 92, 93, 95, 96, 99, 105, 106, 111, 112, 114, 118, 129, 139, 140, 144, 178, 200, 204, 207, 210, 211, 218, 222, 223, 224, 231, 270, 277, 278, 279, 286, 291, 292, 304, 308, 327, 341, 344, 353, 355, 359, 362, 369, 371, 372, 373, 374, 376, 378, 379

Psychiatrist 52

psychological 15, 33, 41, 49, 52, 124, 130, 148, 149, 151, 158, 172, 173, 236, 242, 243, 310, 318, 319, 334, 335, 342, 347, 348, 369, 371

psychosocial 2, 14, 33, 49, 133, 143, 157, 335, 356, 368, 371, 372, 376, 380

Psychosocial 3, 7, 18, 32, 133, 156, 177, 183, 185, 268, 375

Public benefits programs 75

Public Health and Promoting Interoperability Programs 47, 291, 297

Q

QIO 204, 205, 206

QIOs 204

quality 2, 14, 15, 16, 23, 27, 40, 41, 42, 48, 53, 55, 62, 98, 99, 102, 103, 104, 105, 106, 111, 113, 139, 143, 147, 151, 155, 187, 188, 189, 190, 191, 192, 193, 195, 197, 198, 199, 200, 202, 203, 204, 205, 206, 207, 209, 211, 212, 213, 214, 215, 216, 220, 221, 224, 225, 227, 228, 229, 232, 233, 248, 264, 286, 289, 290, 291, 293, 306, 309, 314, 316, 320, 322, 323, 340, 341, 344, 345, 346, 348, 349, 350, 356, 362, 363, 364, 367, 368, 369, 371, 372, 377, 378, 382, 383, 384

Quality iv, 3, 7, 21, 29, 98, 102, 127, 187, 188, 189, 191, 193, 197, 198, 199, 200, 202, 203, 204, 205, 206, 207, 209, 211, 212, 215, 216, 227, 228, 229, 230, 232, 233, 299, 300, 311, 314, 316, 319, 321, 322, 331, 332, 339, 340, 359, 360

quality improvement 104, 106, 188, 190, 192, 193, 195, 200, 203, 205, 212, 214, 228, 229, 232, 356, 382

Quality Improvement Networks (QIN) 204

quality indicators 191, 192, 198, 232

quality management 189, 199, 369

quality measures 98, 204, 207, 215, 291

R

Rancho Los Amigos Scale of Cognitive Functioning 149, 316

Rapid Estimate of Adult Literacy in Medicine (REALM) 146

RCA 276

referral 37, 47, 48, 106, 148, 159, 161, 279, 291, 292, 336, 351, 353, 359, 366, 374

rehabilitation 24, 40, 41, 47, 76, 79, 96, 97, 117, 160, 198, 229, 233, 235, 236, 238, 239, 240, 241, 242, 243, 245, 248, 255, 256, 258, 259, 260, 270, 292, 318, 319, 321, 333, 334, 348, 369, 370, 381

Rehabilitation 3, 7, 68, 97, 116, 117, 197, 198, 229, 233, 235, 236, 238, 239, 240, 241, 248, 254, 255, 259, 260, 261, 319

Reimbursement Methods 3, 7, 13, 59, 123, 267, 290

reimburser 96

religious beliefs 170, 181

reports 21, 27, 209, 214, 215, 216, 217, 309, 325, 340, 342, 353

resource management 14, 16, 349, 354, 362, 369

Resource management 24

resources xv, xvi, xvii, 9, 11, 14, 15, 19, 21, 23, 24, 26, 28, 29, 37, 40, 50, 59, 60, 85, 87, 90, 94, 96, 99, 100, 105, 121, 141, 143, 144, 147, 148, 152, 153, 156, 159, 160, 161, 163, 166, 167, 169, 170, 174, 177, 182, 183, 184, 189, 194, 195, 199, 205, 213, 214, 223, 226, 227, 242, 253, 264, 268, 271, 294, 320, 332, 333, 348, 354, 356, 357, 362, 363, 364, 367, 368, 369, 371, 372, 373, 375, 376, 377, 378, 379, 382, 383

respite 53, 60, 81, 88, 161, 172, 370

retrospective review 115, 127

return on investment 21

reverse mortgage 62

Risk assessment 34, 35, 36, 37, 38, 39

risk management 276

risk sharing 99

Risk stratification 327, 353

root cause 194, 361

Root Cause Analysis (RCA) 276

S

Safety 19, 36, 45, 129, 209, 210, 227, 283, 294, 299, 375

scope of practice 2, 110, 112, 269, 315, 372, 380

screening 17, 18, 32, 129, 148, 150, 165, 183, 208, 224, 287, 335, 353, 371, 372, 374, 375

Screenings 23

Screening tests 38

self-advocacy 23, 143, 144, 182, 372, 382

self-advocate 29

self-efficacy 43, 123, 137, 140, 156, 157, 158, 179, 183, 310, 322, 328, 335, 342, 350, 354, 358

Self-funded plans 71, 313

Self-insured 71

service providers 14, 274, 362, 371, 379, 382

severity 28, 43, 115, 116, 151, 190, 209, 243, 265, 376

Shared decision-making 144

Shared Risk 95

short-term disability (STD) 68

short-term goals 19

Six Sigma 193, 194, 196, 229

Skilled nursing facility 76

SNF 24, 77, 79, 83, 97, 98, 117, 131, 241, 319, 343

social determinants of health 151, 152, 156, 306, 340, 357, 373

Social Security Act 56, 75, 266

What's Next?

Congratulations! You have completed an important part of preparing to sit for your CCM Certification. If you have not already done so, I highly recommend you begin reviewing CCMC's Glossary of Terms. These are the definitions CCMC (the testing organization) uses and they may be different from the definitions where you practice case management.

Although this book and the links to the additional resources have given you a firm foundation for your studies, you may have additional needs. At this point, many people ask about practice tests for the CCM Exam. Although I do not feel they are necessary for everyone, they can play an important role for some. You will find more information on our recommendations for practice tests on the book website.

Some people learn better by hearing information or by having the facts presented in a more conversational tone. If this is you, we offer a popular On-Demand CCM Prep Course. This course is the perfect complement to the book. Where the book gives you the facts, the course brings the facts to life by applying them to case management practice.

For those of you who need accountability and access to an instructor, we offer an Online Live CCM Prep Course three times a year. This course is perfect for those who struggle with studying and need additional support. You have access to the instructors who have helped countless candidates prepare for the CCM Exam. In addition, this course provides you with the accountability necessary to keep moving forward with your studies.

The final step in preparing for your CCM Exam is reviewing our Test Taking Strategies. These are not generic test-taking strategies, but strategies specific to the CCM Exam. They have helped countless candidates pass the CCM Exam, and they will help you too!

More information on all of these resources is available on the book website:

CCMcertificationMadeEasy.com

Made in the USA
Middletown, DE
21 August 2024

59541061R00232